CUTTING AND STYLING
A Salon Handbook

Lesley Hatton
Phillip Hatton
BSc (Hons), MIBiol, CBiol, MIT, MRIPHH, PGCE

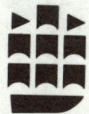

Longman Group Limited,
Longman House, Burnt Mill, Harlow,
Essex, CM20 2JE, England
and Associated Companies throughout the world.

© Lesley Hatton, Phillip Hatton 1987

All rights reserved; no part of this publication may be reproduced, stored in a retrieval system, or transmitted in any form or by any means, electronic, mechanical, photocopying, recording, or otherwise without either the prior written permission of the Publishers or a licence permitting restricted copying in the United Kingdom issued by the Copyright Licensing Agency Ltd, 90 Tottenham Court Road, London, W1P 9HE.

First published 1987
Reprinted 1989
Reprinted with minor amendments 1991
Reprinted by Longman Group Limited 1995

ISBN 0 582 29044 9

British Library Cataloguing in Publication Data
A CIP record for this book is available from the British Library

Produced by Longman Singapore Publishers Pte Ltd
Printed in Singapore

Contents

About this book vi
1 Salon Sense 1
2 Client Communication 24
3 Equipment and Tools 39
4 Design Analysis and Preparation 83
5 Cutting 105
6 Setting and Blow Drying 134
7 Treatments 173
8 Specialised Hair Work 192
9 Salon Organisation 211
Glossary 229
Index 236

About this Book

Like all the Salon Handbooks, *Cutting and Styling* has been written in a direct, easy to understand style. Everyone who works with hair, whether they are experienced hairdressers or trainees, will be able to learn something. Those of you who are at the beginning of your career will get many years of valuable service from this book.

The book deals with a number of different areas of non-chemical work as well as covering areas as diverse as finding your first salon, equipping it, and retailing products. Although there can be no substitute for being shown a practical skill on a one-to-one basis, you will be able to learn many of the skills needed to cut and style hair. There is a section which shows the techniques you will need to work with long hair, a frightening task when you are first confronted with it. If your client has short hair but longs to acquire some longer locks quickly, try hair extensions.

Because clients are our livelihood, we must know exactly what they want before we attempt to give it to them. Even if it is a regular client, pay attention to the tips on analysis before you start working. The non-verbal signals discussed in the book, that your client sends out to you, need to be heeded or you will quickly have an ex-client!

The book is also suitable for anyone taking examinations in hairdressing, whether basic or advanced.

Lesley Hatton
Phillip Hatton

1
Salon Sense

This introductory chapter intended to equip you with relevant knowledge about hair and its chemistry, hygiene and salon safety, and finally the layout of the salon.

1.1 Hair facts

What is hair?

Hair is composed of a type of protein, called keratin. Keratin is different from other proteins because it contains sulphur. It is this sulphur that allows us to perm and straighten hair. Keratin is also a major constituent of our skin and nails, and this is why hairdressing chemicals affect them, as well as the hair for which they were intended. This is why it is sensible always to wear gloves when using chemicals which could otherwise weaken your nails or cause dermatitis.
   Hair is classified into different types:

(1) *Lanugo hair* is found on the human foetus before birth, usually as an unpigmented coat of fine, soft hair. It is shed between the seventh and eighth month of the pregnancy – so we can forget about it as far as hairdressing goes! However, it is always interesting to see how hair develops and changes colour as a baby grows. Some babies have dark hair for the first few months after birth, then it can suddenly change in colour.
(2) *Vellus hair* is the fine downy hair found on the body. If this is dark, some women find its presence embarrassing on the arms, legs, or upper lip because they regard it as a masculine characteristic. It is, however, very

common and considered to be highly sexually attractive in many countries. Excessive hair, or hirsuteness, is often a racial characteristic. (In the British Isles, it is the Welsh who tend to be the most hairy women!) If this hair is bleached, using a product made for such hair, it becomes much less noticeable. A number of chemical hair removers or depilatories are on the market and many women prefer these to shaving because they do not leave any stubble. If you are a women and like to have your legs waxed to remove hair, there is one, sometimes nasty, side-effect – ingrowing hairs! The tip of the newly growing hair cannot penetrate through skin cells which build up across the follicle opening. This results in small spots, often with pus, which contain a coiled hair. Many women use needles to remove them before they get painful, but be careful to use sterile needles (clean them with alcohol or disinfectant). It is better to leave the hair in place (work it free rather than remove it) so that the skin will leave an exit for the hair above the follicle. If you remove the hair the skin will heal over completely and the ingrowing hair will recur. As prevention is better than cure, scrub your legs with a mild abrasive such as a Buf-Puf or loofah each time you bath or shower. This will remove the dead skin which otherwise blocks the follicle opening. This should be carried out a few days after waxing.

(3)   *Terminal hair* is the hair hairdressers are concerned with. It is coarser than vellus hair and is found on the scalp, on men's faces, under the arms, and on the pubic areas. Terminal facial and body hair is under the control of the male hormones – the androgens – which start to be secreted at puberty by the testes in males. Women also secrete these male hormones, although in a much weaker form, from the adrenal glands. Without these hormones neither men nor women would get pubic or underarm hair!

Unfortunately, a number of women have trouble as they get older, with facial hairs becoming coarser. This is due to the effect of the hormonal changes associated with the 'change of life', and if the hair is unsightly it is best to have it removed by electrolysis. This may require several treatments, but is the only really effective permanent method of hair removal.

How does a hair grow?

A hair grows from a minute pit in the skin called a hair follicle. The hair that we see emerging from the scalp is dead, but at the base of the follicle the hair is alive and actively growing. At the base of the follicle, in the area most hairdressers refer to as the bulb, is a group of cells called the papilla. It is in this papilla that cells undergo a type of cell division called *mitosis*. During this division two exact copies of a cell are made. Cells are constantly dividing and pushing upwards, changing into different areas of the hair until they die and have keratin laid down inside them. All this occurs in the bottom third of the follicle. As the hair we see is dead, we cannot alter how it grows by any hairdressing process or treatment. Cutting does not alter the speed of growth or the diameter of the hair. Thus the story of shaving legs making the hairs grow coarser is untrue. Many young men who shave for the first time are convinced that shaving has made their beards coarser, but it is only because recently shaved stubble feels coarser than if a beard is left to grow (simply because of the length of the hair). The saying that regular haircuts make your hair grow faster is also untrue.

Once a hair has been damaged, it cannot be permanently repaired. It is possible to mask the damage with special conditioners, but the only way to change the quality of the hair permanently is through diet, since food and oxygen get into the hair through the blood supply to the dividing cells of the papilla.

This is why the hairdresser must be fully aware of the potential damage that can be caused to hair by the various hairdressing chemicals and treatments that are used. Clients see the hairdresser as a professional person who knows what he or she is doing and what is best for their hair. Make sure that their faith is properly placed. You can advise them about washing their hair, conditioning it, and how to maintain a style. All of these can bring the salon extra business as well as creating happier clients, who appreciate that you are taking an interest in them.

What is the structure of a hair like?

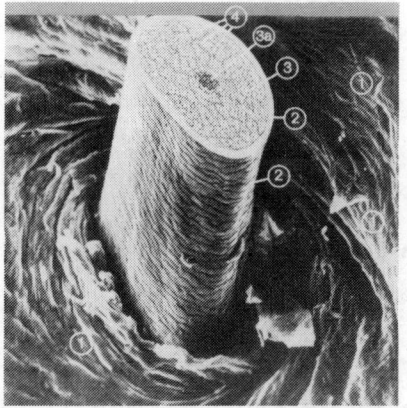

Fig. 1.1 The hair shaft emerging from the scalp.
(1) The horny layer of epidermis which can be seen around the follicle opening.
(2) The cuticle, showing the various overlapping layers of scales.
(3) The columnar cortical cells that contain granules of pigment.
(3a) The medulla, a series of air spaces in the centre of the hair.
(4) The intracellular cement that surrounds the cortical fibres. (Reproduced courtesy of Wella Ltd.)

Figure 1.1 shows a highly magnified hair emerging from a hair follicle. It was taken by research scientists who work for Wella in Germany, using an electron microscope. The scales that you can see are one of several layers (about seven in European hair, and up to eleven in Chinese hair). This outer layer is known as the cuticle. There are more cuticle layers around the hair shaft near the base of the hair than there are towards the older tip of the hair, purely because of wear and tear. It is the protective layer of the hair and prevents substances from entering the layers below. The cuticle is rather like the tiles on a roof which protect a house from the weather. But unlike a roof, there are several layers.

These layers are sometimes held together by small 'press studs', giving an extremely strong connection between neighbouring layers of cuticle. In Fig. 1.2 these studs can clearly be seen in the top right-hand corner of the photograph. In this particular photograph some seven cuticle layers can be counted. The free ends of the overlapping scales (called imbrications) point upwards in the direction of the hair growth, that is, towards the tip. If you take a hair between the finger and thumb and gently rub it up and down the hair, you will find it feels smooth from root to point, but rough from point to root. This is because the tips of the cuticle scales cause resistance. As the cuticle scales are translucent (allowing some light to pass through them) we can see the colour of the hair in the layer below.

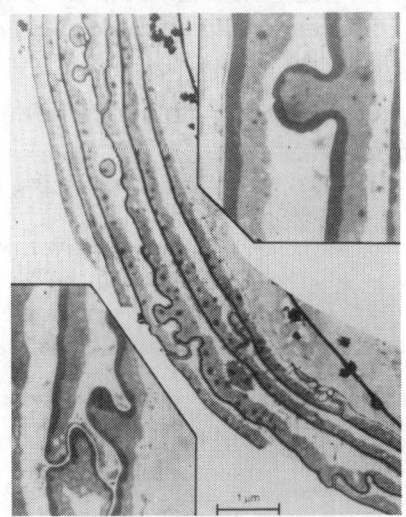

Fig. 1.2 The overlapping cuticle scales of human hair which are held together by a cellular cement and mechanical 'press studs'.
(Reproduced courtesy of Wella Ltd.)

If the cuticle is damaged by excessive physical or chemical treatment, the second layer of the hair, the cortex, may be exposed to injury. This second layer forms the bulk of the hair and it is in this part that permanent chemical changes take place: perming, straightening, bleaching and tinting.

The cortex is the most important layer of the hair and makes up between 75 per cent to 90 per cent of the hairs' bulk. It contains the natural pigment of the hair (mostly melanin if the hair is black to brown or mostly pheomelanin if the hair is yellow to red). This pigment is produced at the bottom of the follicle by a cell called a melanocyte. If the melanocyte should stop working, no colour is produced and the hair becomes white. If there is a mixture of white and coloured hairs on the scalp an illusion of greyness results. There is, however, no such thing as an individual grey hair – try plucking one!

Many of the physical properties of hair are dependent on the cortex. These include:

- strength;
- elasticity;
- direction and types of growth (straight, curly);
- diameter of the hair shaft;

Put simply, the cortex has a structure rather like a bunch of straws (called macrofibrils) which are held together by a network of keratin fibres. Within each of the 'straws' are finer tubes (called microfibrils), which contain a group of three coiled polypeptide chains (known as the protofibril). These chains have a spiral shape called an alpha-helix, and look rather like a spiral staircase. These polypeptide chains are like springs held together by ladder-like cross-linkages. These chains give the hair its elasticity, enabling it to be stretched, yet still spring back to its original length. Keratin in its normal unstretched state is called alpha-keratin. When stretched it forms beta-keratin, which should spring back to alpha-keratin once pressure is taken off the hair. The entire structure is held together by various types of bonds, with the surrounding cuticle forming a tough protective outer coat.

The centre of the hair is the medulla. More nonsense has been said about this than any other part of the hair. It is basically an air space, which may contain melanin. Some people have a medulla throughout the length of each hair, some have one only in parts of each hair, and some have none at all – while others have two! As it serves no useful purpose, ignore it!

1.2 Hair chemistry

Keratin — the protein

As has already been mentioned, hair is made of a type of protein called keratin. Proteins are complex organic (meaning that they contain carbon) compounds which all contain carbon, hydrogen, oxygen and nitrogen. Keratin contains these four elements as well as sulphur. Proteins make up about 12 per cent of the weight of the human body and are needed for growth and replacement of body cells. Because nitrogen cannot be stored by the body a daily intake is necessary if growth is to be normal.

All proteins are made up of small amino acids. There are about twenty-two different types of amino acid and they can be arranged in any order to make up a protein.

Each amino acid is joined end-on-end like a series of bricks in a wall. They are held together by peptide or end-bonds. These strings of amino acids held together by their peptide bonds are known as polypeptides (the prefix 'poly' on a word means many). Polypeptides in long coiled chains may contain many hundreds of amino acids and are sometimes referred to as 'simple' proteins. More complicated proteins are formed when adjacent spirals of polypeptides are cross-linked by other bonds. Human hair is called a 'fibre' protein and it possesses an exceptional number of cross-bonds or linkages.

Cross-linkages of hair

There are three types of cross-linkage in the keratin of hair, illustrated in Fig. 1.3.

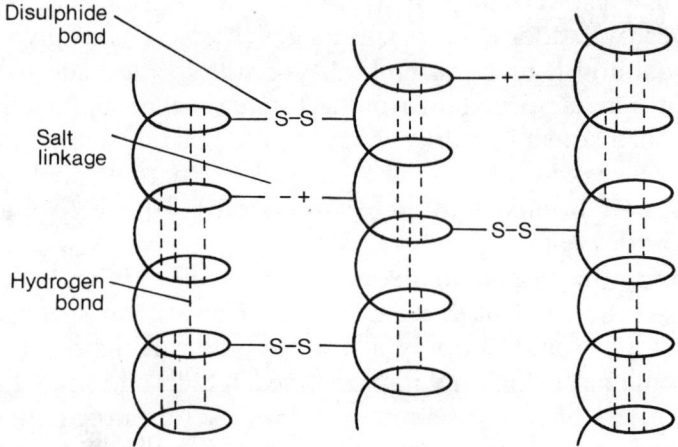

Fig. 1.3 The three types of cross-linkage found in keratin.

(1) *Disulphide linkages*. These are the most important bonds as far as perming and straightening are concerned as it is these that are broken to allow the alteration of the hair shape. The amino acid cystine forms a link through its central disulphide bond between two adjacent polypeptide chains. It is this cystine or disulphide linkage that we were referring to earlier when we said that the linkages were like rungs of a ladder. These are very strong bonds which can be broken only by chemicals.

Average hair contains between 4–5 per cent sulphur, but natural red hair may contain up to 8 per cent sulphur. Because this is almost twice as much as in normal hair, red hair, with its higher sulphur content, is more resistant and difficult to perm.

(2) *Salt linkages.* The amino acids that form polypeptides may have free acid (negative) or basic amino (positive) groups. If a free negative charge in one polypeptide chain lies opposite a free positive charge in an adjacent chain there will be an attraction between them. Opposite electrical charges attract, rather like the North and South poles of a magnet. These salt linkages are also called ionic or electrostatic charges. Because they are weaker than the disulphide linkages they can be easily broken by weak acids or alkalis. If you quickly run a nylon comb through your hair for a minute it will be able to attract and pick up a small piece of paper. The comb has picked up a charge from the hair and the opposite charge induced in the piece of paper attracts the two together. This is an example of an electrostatic charge.

(3) *Hydrogen bonds.* These weak bonds are due to the attraction between hydrogen atoms and oxygen atoms (like the salt linkage this is an electrostatic attraction). This can occur in a polypeptide chain (between the coils) or between adjacent polypeptide chains. Since they form cross-bonds, they help the disulphide bonds to keep adjacent polypeptide chains together, giving 'body' to the hair. Although the hydrogen bonds are very weak, many more of them are present than any other bond in the hair. They can be broken by water and most weak chemicals, and will be discussed fully in Chapter 6, *Setting and Blow Drying.*

Free amino acids

Between the chains of keratin in the cortex of the hair are found 'free' amino acids. These do not appear to play any structural role but help to hold moisture within the cortex. The level of moisture is maintained at about 10 per cent by the amino acids and the coating of sebum on the cuticle. Moisture is important to keep the hair pliable.

In hair where the cuticle is damaged, shampooing can remove some of the free amino acids. The level of moisture in the cortex falls and the condition of the hair suffers. To counteract this some treatments contain free amino acids or treated protein.

1.3 All about pH

What is pH?

The term 'pH' is simply a way of indicating how acid or alkaline something is. pH is expressed on a scale from 0 to 14, with 7.0 in the middle being the

8 Cutting and Styling: a salon handbook

neutral point, where something is neither acid or alkaline. A simple pH scale is shown in Fig. 1.4.

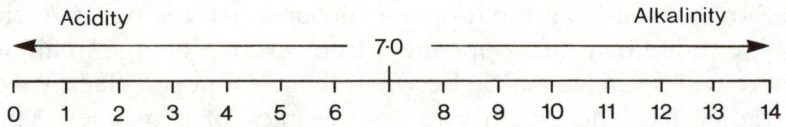

Fig. 1.4 A simple pH scale to show acidity and alkalinity.

Why is pH important?

pH is important because of the way it affects the hair. Acids close (remember *c* for close) the cuticle of the hair, leaving it shiny and manageable. The natural pH of the skin and hair ranges between 4.5 – 5.5 because of this, and because this pH also inhibits the growth of bacteria. Hair in its acid state resists processing. Alkaline chemicals open the cuticle of the hair and cause the hair shaft to swell. This is important to allow the entry of chemicals into the cortex (tints, bleaches and cold perms). Hair in an alkaline state will facilitate processing. However, a high pH (usually above 10) can destroy the structure of hair. Such chemicals are called depilatories and are sold to remove unwanted hair on legs and other parts of the body.

What is a 'pH-balanced' product?

This is simply a product that has the same pH as the hair and skin, approximately 5. Such products will not upset the natural pH. After many alkaline hairdressing treatments, acid rinses are used to bring the pH back to its normal level.

How do I test pH?

One way is to use litmus, which will be red in acids and blue in alkalis. Litmus is available as paper or a liquid. It has the disadvantage that it can only tell you if a chemical is acid or alkaline, not how weak or strong it is. The second way is to use universal indicator, and this changes over a range of colours corresponding to different pHs. The colour is simply matched up to a chart. Universal indicator is available as paper or liquid.

1.4 Hygiene in the salon

Why is hygiene important in the salon?

Following certain routines of hygiene will help prevent the possible spread of infection. Never before have hairdressers and beauty therapists been so concerned about the risk of spreading infection during their work. This concern has much to do with the arrival on the scene of the HIV virus that causes AIDS.

For years, however, it has been possible to contract a variety of other diseases during a visit to the hairdresser, though these, of course, were not killers. It is important that the industry is seen to be doing its fair share to protect clients. Many salons do not know what to do, so we will make some suggestions for guidelines. Although the public are most concerned about AIDS, these guidelines will also help to prevent other diseases such as hepatitis, impetigo, and ringworm.

Is the client in any danger from the hairdresser?

The simple answer is 'yes', but only if the hairdresser has an infectious disease. The golden rule should be that you do not touch a client if you have some kind of infectious skin condition yourself, unless this is on the body and is covered by clothes. If you have something wrong with you, ask your doctor if it is necessary to take precautions to stop it spreading. Remember that there are many skin conditions, such as dandruff and psoriasis, which cannot be caught. For further reading on non-infectious conditions, see *Hygiene – A Salon Handbook*.

How can dangers be minimised for the client?

- You should wash your hands if you have been to the toilet, sneezed, blown your nose, or eaten something.
- Always use sterile tools on each client, including fresh towels.
- Where possible use disposable neck-strips, etc.
- Check the head of every client before you shampoo. Check for possible infections, or infestations of lice. Be suspicious if the skin is at all red or scratched. Working on a client with an infectious condition puts other clients at risk.
- Wash down salon surfaces as a regular routine.
- Keep bins covered and use pedal type if possible.

10 Cutting and Styling: a salon handbook

What methods are suitable to sterilise tools in the salon?

The words 'sterilise' and 'disinfect' have slightly differing meanings. If you sterilise anything, it will become completely free of all living organisms. Disinfectants will kill germs if used long enough and strong enough. Many people will not carry out the process of disinfection correctly, and it is possible that some resistant spores will survive. In salons it is important always to clean a piece of equipment before any method of sterilisation is carried out. You cannot sterilise dirty equipment, so before using any of the methods described below, wash your equipment in hot soapy water.

(a) Moist heat sterilisation involves boiling water, so is only suitable for equipment that can withstand heat or which will not rust. Towels should be washed between every client, and the hot wash cycle of most washing machines should be suitable for this. It is designated as wash cycle 1 and should reach 95°C. Boiling water can be used to sterilise some heat-resistant plastics but the problems associated with steam and condensation must be considered. It is possible to cause electrical safety hazards if there is excessive condensation, and it is always irritating if mirrors steam up. One of the most effective methods of sterilisation is with an autoclave, a sophisticated type of pressure cooker. By trapping steam inside a sealed vessel so that there is a build-up of pressure, the boiling point of water can be increased from 100°C to 121°C, ensuring sterilisation. This is illustrated in Fig. 1.5. Some manufacturers are trying to develop electrically operated autoclaves that can be bought cheaply and operated without danger in salons. Between 20–30 minutes is required for moist heat to be effective.

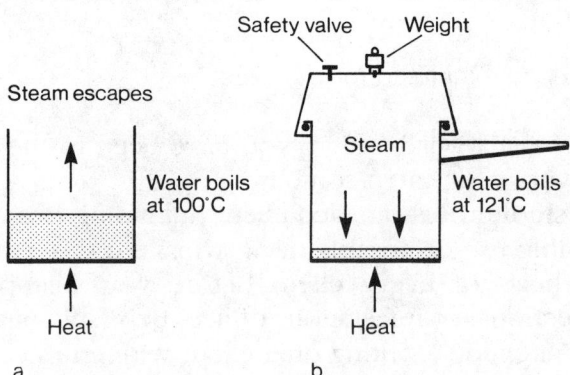

Fig. 1.5 Water boiling (a) in an open container and (b) in a pressure cooker.

(b) Chemical vapour. This method involves the use of a cabinet that allows equipment to be surrounded by a sterilising vapour. The vapour

used is formaldehyde, which is produced by placing some liquid formalin in a dish above an electrically operated heater. Once the formalin is heated it gives off the formaldehyde vapour. The cabinet has perforated metal shelving for equipment to be placed on. A diagram of a cabinet is shown in Fig. 1.6. It is particularly useful for hair nets and sponges, as the vapour will penetrate them. It is not recommended for metal tools as it attacks the surface and can cause pitting. Use for 20 minutes. There have been scares about formaldehyde causing cancer, but if used as directed a cabinet should be safe.

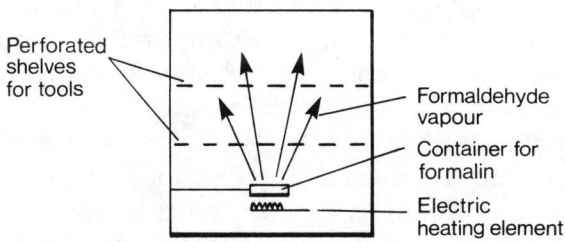

Fig. 1.6 Formaldehyde cabinet.

(c) Ultra-violet radiation. This is used in many salons in sterilising cabinets. It is frequently used because it looks modern and does not produce smells. It is effective only on the surfaces that the ultra-violet rays touch, so is not suitable for equipment that needs more than surface sterilisation. Tools must be turned because the mercury vapour lamp that produces the ultra-violet light is situated at the top of the cabinet, as shown in Figure 1.7. These cabinets are good places to keep tools which have been sterilised by other methods until they are ready for use.

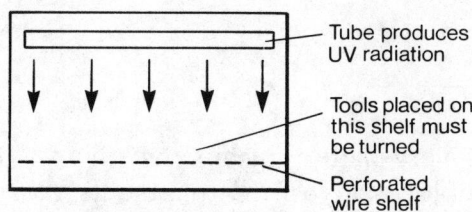

Fig. 1.7 Ultra-violet sterilising cabinet.

(d) Disinfectants. A variety of disinfectants is on the market and manufacturers are marketing products which are specifically for use in salons. Because your tools are in constant use, disinfecting jars such as the

ones produced by Barbicide are particularly useful. Tools can be stored in the disinfectant, in this case a quaternary ammonium compound, in between clients. Barbicide was first patented in America by a chemist who had picked up ringworm while at the hairdresser! Figure 1.8 shows jars in two sizes. The one on the left is designed for manicure equipment, while the one on the right is for hairdressing tools. This particular solution will not cause rusting so is particularly suitable for scissors, razors, clipper blades, brushes and combs. The tools can be removed from the Barbicide jar by raising the lid as shown by the jar on the right.

Some other suitable disinfectants are available, based on compounds such as glutaraldehyde which are equally effective. Alcohol can also be used to sterilise your tools, but remember that this is flammable so should never be used near a naked flame. The most important point about using disinfectants is to make up solutions freshly as directed by the manufacturer. Clean your tools before immersing them in the solution, leave them in the *required* time and change solutions as directed by the manufacturer. Check with the manufacturer about rusting of metal tools before you commit your salon to using a particular brand. Remember also to wash down work surfaces daily, with hot soapy water and disinfectant. Never use abrasive cleaners for cleaning surfaces (including basins) as these will cause tiny scratch marks where germs can multiply.

After sterilisation is complete (by whatever method), equipment will only remain sterile until it comes into contact with the air in the salon. Keep it in a sterilisation cabinet until its next use. Do not place tools in pockets, or hold clips in the mouth, or place equipment on dirty worksurfaces.

1.5 Salon safety

Hairdressing, by its very nature, means that there is bound to be close contact with the public. Many of the treatments carried out in the salon could cause damage to the hair and skin of the client. Before carrying out chemical treatments you should therefore carry out precautionary tests first. These are fully explained in *Colouring – A Salon Handbook* and *Perming and Straightening – A Salon Handbook*. What we are concerned with here is general salon safety, so that the risk of accidents is minimised for clients and salon employees. Under the 1974 Health and Safety at Work

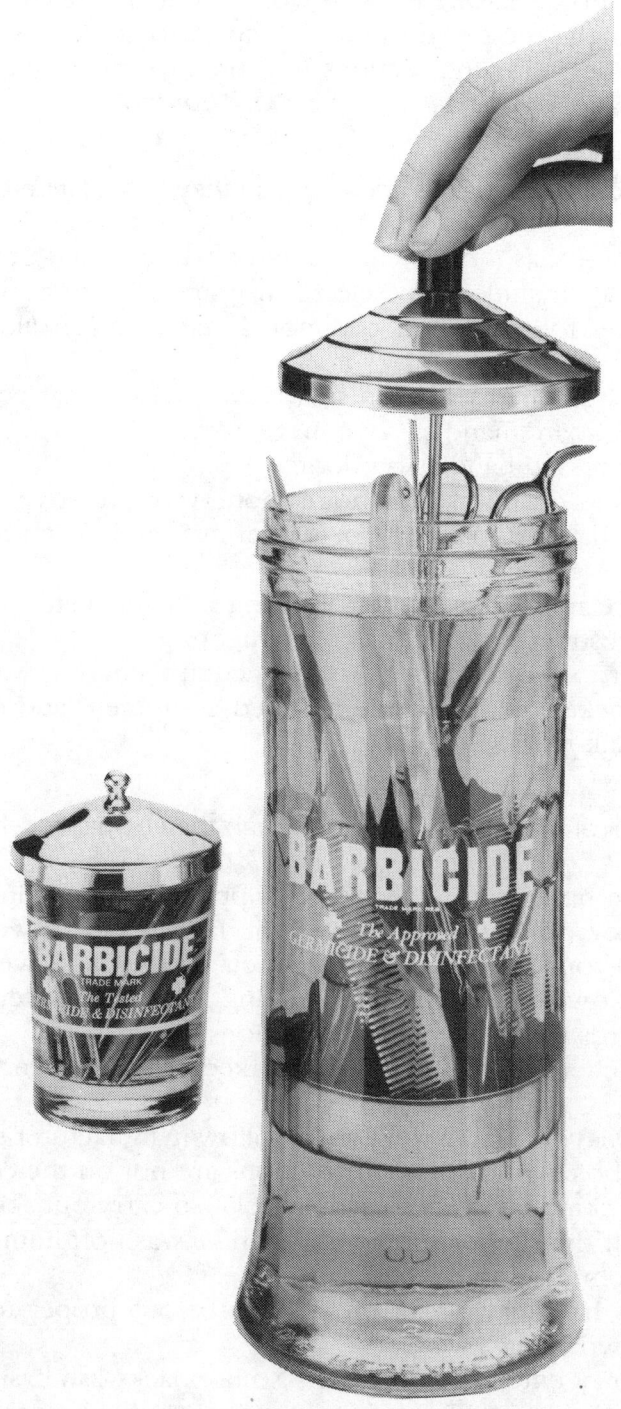

Fig. 1.8 Barbicide disinfecting jars being used on a variety of tools. (Courtesy of Renscene Ltd.)

Act, it is your duty to ensure the safety of the public while they are in the salon. Interestingly, these regulations also apply to home or self-employed hairdressers. The following sections are intended as a quick guide; for further information see *Hygiene – A Salon Handbook*.

What are physical salon hazards and how can they be minimised?

The average salon has a number of hazards which could be classified as physical. These include the salon furniture, flooring, lighting and equipment. The following are common hazards, given alongside their remedies.

People may hurt themselves on sharp edges and square corners, or on protruding cupboard handles – so have rounded corners on all work surfaces and recessed handles on doors.

Shoes may slip on floors which are slippery or are covered with spilt liquids – so have non-slip floor coverings and wipe up spillages immediately.

Accidents are most likely where lighting is inadequate, through poor visibility or eyestrain, so install adequate lighting.

People may trip on trailing wires or over equipment near walk-ways – so install more sockets or have wall-mounted equipment and do not leave anything in walk-ways.

What are chemical salon hazards and how can they be minimised?

Chemical salon hazards are due to the inappropriate handling and use of chemicals. They can cause damage to the hairdresser as well as clients. Always gown your clients to protect their clothes and wear gloves to protect your own hands when handling chemicals. Here are some common hazards followed by their solutions:

The wrong chemical may be used – so keep chemicals in their original bottles.

A chemical may be used wrongly – so follow manufacturer's instructions and keep the boxes in case the instructions are not on the containers.

The client's skin may react to a chemical – so carry out skin test before use *or* keep off the skin *or* protect the skin *or* wash off immediately (you may need a combination of these).

The client's hair may break off – so carry out proper testing *before* commencing work.

Chemicals may enter a client's eye – so use backwash basins *or* change cotton wool strips regularly *or* do not apply too much chemical.

A chemical may catch fire – so do not have a naked flame near chemicals!

Someone may begin to cough badly when a chemical is in the air – so try to direct hairspray away from that person, ensure adequate ventilation, and wear a mask when you are preparing powder bleach.

What are electrical salon hazards and how can they be minimised?

Every salon must have electricity. It must be used safely or a fatal injury could occur in the salon. These are guidelines which should be followed:

- All electrical equipment should have a British Standards number to show that it is safe to use.
- Appliances should be fitted with a correctly wired plug, protected by the right size of fuse.
- Have one plug to each socket outlet – never use adaptors or you may overload sockets.
- Never handle electrical appliances with wet hands and do not use them near water.
- If a plug is broken or an appliance lead is damaged replaced them.

> If in doubt, consult an electrician

What could cause a fire in the salon?

Salons contain chemicals which are flammable (setting lotions, hair sprays, styling aids) and others which support combustion should a fire occur (peroxide-based products). For this reason, store flammable products away from peroxide. Fires are most likely if salons have heating which relies on gas, electrical or paraffin fires. Anything place in front of such fires could ignite. Central heating will eliminate this cause. Adequate ashtrays should always be provided for smokers. Never use naked flames in the salon when, for example, attaching hair extensions.

What action should be taken in the event of a fire?

- Get clients out of the salon.
- If time permits, close doors and windows to starve the fire of oxygen and stop it spreading so quickly.
- Phone for the fire brigade as quickly as possible.

- Tackle a small fire with the salon fire extinguisher by aiming at the sides or base of the fire (never use water-type extinguishers on electrical fires).

1.6 Salon layout

The overall planning and design of the salon premises is very important to how well a salon runs, to the type of customer it attracts, and the prices that can be charged.

If the salon is badly designed and under-equipped the staff will not be able to work as effectively as they otherwise could. There must be adequate styling positions, driers, basins and other equipment to cope with the peak number of customers in the salon, not the minimum. If a customer has not got much time each week for a salon visit she will resent unnecessary delays.

Competition between salons is never-ending, and you must endeavour to develop and then maintain attractive, yet safe, surroundings in the salon.

Salon designs and colour schemes have become trademarks of some of the larger salon chains. The design can be repeated around the country so that the same 'image' is conveyed wherever the salon is situated. We can all learn a great deal from the 'flagships' of the industry. What they have spent thousands of pounds on developing with professional designers can yield good ideas which can be copied on a smaller scale. If you are on holiday abroad, check the salons; you never know what you might see. Like it or not, first appearances count. You will attract more clients into the salon in the first place if it looks a pleasant place to be.

General salon layout

It wasn't that long ago that clients had their hair done in the privacy of an individual cubicle! Each was fitted with a basin, drier, styling unit, etc. The client could keep an appointment by seeing only one member of staff and none of the other clients. The salon of today is based on the 'open-plan' style. Certain areas being designated for particular services such as tinting and perming, drying, and a bank of basins or 'wet' area.

Colour scheme

The overall colour scheme is vital in creating the right atmosphere and congenial working conditions. For example, walls painted bright red will cast a warm glow onto the hair, giving a deceptive warmth to hair colours. Alternatively, dark blue walls have the opposite effect, casting cool shadows which kill warmth. The best colours for walls are soft, pastel shades which will be neutral in their effect on hair colour. Have strong colour in areas where it will not affect the colour judgement of hair, such as the reception. Wherever possible, use washable materials so that walls can be easily cleaned. This will make redecoration less frequent in the future!

Lighting

Lighting must be adequate to prevent accidents. Direct glare can cause eyestrain and should be eliminated with plastic or glass diffusers. These 'soften' the light. Having ordinary tungsten filament light bulbs can cause a yellow cast on hair, so should be avoided as this type of light will give a false impression of colour results. The nearest thing to daylight is 'warm white' fluorescent lighting. It will give an even illumination so is recommended to avoid eyestrain. If you wish to enhance the look of hair, cleverly placed spotlights can make the hair shine. If you ever go to a colour demonstration the hairdresser will usually show off the finished head under a spotlight. Take this apparently shiny head under some flourescent lights and it will appear much flatter. Using a mixture of such lighting is the answer.

Flooring

Because of the nature of the work in a salon it is a good idea to have floors which are washable. Sheet vinyl is good for this as it will not lift up at the edges, like tiles. It can be non-slip as well, which gives an added safety bonus. If carpet is used anywhere in the general salon area it must be firmly fixed so people cannot trip. It would also be wise to have a hard-wearing carpet where people walk so that some parts do not wear quicker than others. Choose a washable material as well.

Styling Units

Styling units can either be the 'island' type that sit in the middle of the floor, or they can be fixed along the walls of the salon. Some narrow salons will be forced to have the latter, but if the salon is wide enough, islands can create extra working space.

Figure 1.9 shows a typical modern salon with styling units along one side of a wall. There is space for a trolley alongside each unit, adequate

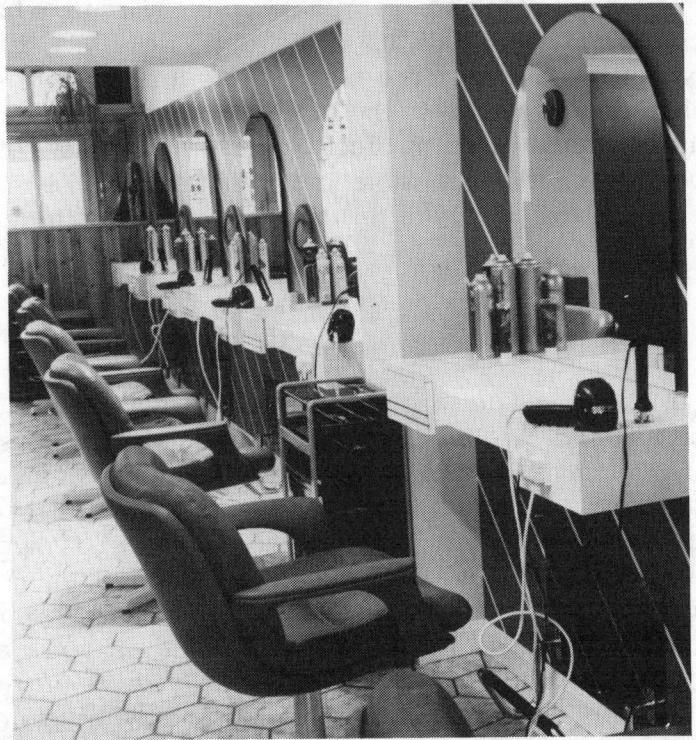

Fig. 1.9 A set of styling units fixed along a salon wall. (Courtesy of Pietranera (UK) Ltd.)

electrical power, individual mirrors and space to place products and equipment. Make sure that the units you choose have storage space for your hairdrier in the form of a hole in the work surface or a hook to hang it from. A hole for hot tongs to be placed in has been provided on this particular unit, which will help eliminate accidents. Notice, as well, how the wall is protected from marking by the foot rest and shielding. This will help lengthen the working life of your decorations and make the client comfortable if the chairs do not have their own footrests.

Heating and Ventilation

It is important to keep the salon temperature around 20°C (68°F), because clients with wet hair can feel the cold as the moisture evaporates from their hair. The best form of heating is some form of central heating, because radiators can be fixed to walls where they present no hazard and the temperature can be kept constant by thermostats.

Ventilation is important to keep the composition of the air constant. There should not be a build-up of water vapour or stale air, which will make clients and staff alike feel uncomfortable. Ventilation does not just mean opening a window so there is a blast of fresh air! This would make a client with wet hair feel cold. If windows are opened, they should be louvred or the hopper type, so that incoming air can be directed towards the ceiling so that it can first be warmed up. The air in a salon should be changed about three times an hour. The amount of air to be changed can be calculated by multiplying the height of the salon ceiling by its width and then its length. This figure is the cubic capacity or volume of the salon, and if this is multiplied by three it will give the air change per hour. Electrical extractor fans can be used to achieve such air changes in a controlled manner. When you have them installed, check their rating per hour for extracting air, and use either one large fan or a couple of smaller ones to extract enough air. The siting of fans is important. Do not place near an air inlet such as an open window or door, or you will simply extract fresh air. Siting one near sources of moisture (drier banks and basins) can help eliminate condensation. In hot weather good ventilation will also help a salon to feel cooler.

1.7 First aid

It is extremely important for everyone who deals with the general public to have some knowledge of first aid, especially when offering a service where accidents could happen.

First aid is the first action that should be taken to minimise damage in the case of an accident or sudden illness. It is discussed fully, with reasons for the actions taken, in *Hygiene – A Salon Handbook* but here is a quick reference for the more common emergencies you may encounter.

Bleeding

In the event of a minor cut apply pressures with the fingers until bleeding stops. Use alum powder in men's hairdressing, (Don't use a styptic pencil because of the risk of cross-infection.) If there is a large loss of blood, apply pressure using clean towels or the hands and phone for an ambulance. In the case of a nose bleed, pinch the soft part of the nose, lean the head forward and do not blow the nose for some time afterwards.

Burns

Whether burns are dry or wet (scalds), cool the skin immediately by immersing in cold running water. If you cannot get a client to water hold a soaking wet towel against the damaged area. Seek medical advice if the burn is large. A large burn can be covered with sterile gauze until medical help arrives. If a chemical burn occurs, flood the area with water. In the eye it is better to use flowing water rather than an eye bath.

Fainting

If a client feels faint, put his or her head down between the knees and loosen tight clothing. If a client has fainted, raise his or her legs on a cushion so that they are higher than the head. Using smelling salts will shock someone out of a faint but do nothing to alleviate the cause; for this reason we do not recommend smelling salts.

Hysterical fit

This occurs when someone has lost control of his or her emotions. It should be treated by getting the person alone (away from an audience), being firm and not expressing sympathy. After the hysteria has died away do not express sympathy as the client may start again.

Epileptic fit

Many people who suffer from epilepsy are on medication which reduces the chance of fits occurring. If a fit does occur, however, the client will fall unconscious to the floor. After a short period of time, the limbs will begin to jerk uncontrollably. When this happens make sure that any objects that can cause injury are removed. After the fit, lay the client in the recovery position (on one side) so that he or she cannot choke or smother on vomit. It is usual to phone an ambulance if it is someone you do not know.

Breathing stops

For whatever reason this occurs, check the airways to see if they are blocked. if they are, tilt the head back to unblock them. Now begin mouth to mouth resuscitation by covering the mouth with yours. While squeezing the nostrils together, blow into the mouth. The chest will rise and then fall. Repeat until breathing resumes and ask someone else to phone for an ambulance (by continuing mouth to mouth resuscitation you are preventing possible brain damage).

Heart attack

The client may complain of chest pains and the skin may go blue. In this case keep the client upright and loosen the clothing. If the client is on the floor, support the back on cushions to prop him or her up. If the heart stops, begin mouth to mouth resuscitation and alternate this with cardiac massage (press firmly down once on the breast bone). Check for a pulse and get someone to phone for an ambulance.

Electric shock

If someone is being electrocuted do not touch them but try to turn off the electricity. Do this by unplugging at the mains or by turning the switches off. If the heart stops begin mouth to mouth resuscitation and cardiac massage until the patient recovers.

Fractures

Keep the patient still if you suspect a broken bone (a leg or arm may be at a peculiar angle). Phone for an ambulance.

> Never give alcohol to anyone who is feeling ill or who has been hurt in case they should need an anaesthetic on entry to hospital.

The first aid box

All salons should have a first aid box which is available in the event of an accident. This requirement varies with the number of people on the premises and is governed by the Health and Safety (First Aid) Regulations of 1982. The first aid box should be marked with a red cross on a white background *or* a white cross on a red background *or* a white cross on a green background. The box should close tightly so that it is dust- and moisture-free. It should be put in a place that all employees are aware of.

22 Cutting and Styling: a salon handbook

Item in first aid box	Minimum no. of items required	
	1–10 employees	11–50 employees
First aid guidance card	1	1
Individual sterile plasters	20	40
Medium sterile dressings	2	4
Large sterile dressings	2	4
Extra large sterile dressings	2	4
Sterile eye pads/bandage	2	4
Triangular bandages/slings	2	4
Sterilised wound coverings	2	4
Safety pins	6	12

These are the minimum recommended contents. It is useful to have some liquid and cream disinfectant/antiseptic; cotton wool and tissues; surgical adhesive tape; a crepe bandage for a sprain and a bowl for pouring water. The first things to run out in a first aid box are plasters. As it makes sense to keep cuts covered, have a supply of waterproof ones for protection.

1.8 Questions

1. What is hair composed of?
2. Why is this different from other proteins?
3. Why should you wear gloves when handling chemicals?
4. What is lanugo hair?
5. What is vellus hair?
6. How would you remove or disguise unwanted hair?
7. What is terminal hair on the body influenced by?
8. What is the only permanent method of hair removal?
9. Where does the hair grow from?
10. How does cutting alter hair growth?
11. Why can't damaged hair be permanently repaired?
12. How many layers of cuticle has a hair?
13. What does 'translucent' mean?
14. What properties of hair are dependent on the cortex?
15. What are alpha- and beta-keratin?
16. Why do you need a daily intake of protein in your diet?
17. Name the three types of cross-linkage found in keratin.
18. Why are free amino acids important to hair?
19. What does pH measure?

20 Why does hair in an acid state resist processing?
21 Why does hair in an alkaline state facilitate processing?
22 How could you test the pH of a chemical?
23 Why is hygiene important in the salon?
24 List ways in which you can prevent infection spreading in the salon.
25 Describe two methods of sterilising using moist heat.
26 How do you sterilise using chemical vapours?
27 How and when would you use an ultra-violet cabinet?
28 What precautions would you take when using disinfectants to sterilise tools?
29 Describe some physical salon hazards and how they can be minimised.
30 Describe some chemical salon hazards and how they can be minimised.
31 Describe some electrical safety precautions that you would always observe.
32 What kinds of things could result in the outbreak of fire in a salon and what would you do in the event of a fire?
33 Why is salon layout important for business?
34 What types of lighting would you put in a salon?
35 Give reasons for the type of flooring you might place in a salon.
36 Why might you use island style styling units?
37 What should a good styling unit have incorporated into it?
38 Why is central heating ideal for salons?
39 Give reasons for installing adequate ventilation.
40 What is the purpose of first aid?
41 What is the first aid for bleeding?
42 What is the first aid for a burn?
43 Why is flowing water best to use if a chemical enters the eye?
44 Give the first aid if a client feels faint or has fainted.
45 What is the first aid for an hysterical fit?
46 What action would you take in the event of a client having an epileptic fit?
47 What is the first aid if someone should stop breathing?
48 If someone has a heart attack what should you do?
49 If someone is being electrocuted why should you not touch them?
50 If a client fell and you suspected a fracture, what action would you take?
51 What items should be found in every first aid box?
52 Why should a first aid box be easy to identify?
53 What items are likely to run out first from a first aid box?

2 Client Communication

The most successful salons are the ones which succeed in attracting *and keeping* clients. No matter how much money and talent has been spent on decoration, it is the attitude and professionalism of the staff that will keep the clients. If a client is attracted by the decor but does not return, there is usually something wrong with the service. This could be dissatisfaction with the result of her hair, or simply the way she has been dealt with. Going to the hairdresser should be the treat of the week, making the client not only feel good, but feel positive about herself (or himself) as well.

2.1 What do clients expect from a visit to the salon?

Listed below are examples of what clients usually expect from a visit to the salon:

- a good cut;
- a manageable style;
- friendliness;
- prompt and attentive personal service;
- hair advice;
- pleasant surroundings;
- a high standard of hygiene;
- professionalism.

How does your salon score on these points? You can probably think of a lot more examples to add to the above list. It is important to maintain the same level of service from the moment the client enters the salon until the moment they leave.

2.2 The reception

The first contact a client has with a salon is when she makes her appointment. There are two ways of doing this:

(a) by telephoning the salon;
(b) by visiting the salon.

First impressions count. Her first encounter of the salon, whether by telephone or in person, should give her a good impression. If it is unfavourable, you may lose the client before an appointment is even kept!

In larger salons this problem is often overcome by employing a full-time receptionist. They will deal with answering the phone, making appointments, cash transactions, and generally organising the flow of clients in and out of the salon. In salons where this is not possible, all the staff will act at some time as the receptionist, as and when required. For this reason it is important that all salon staff are conversant and practised in the operations of the reception area, so that a uniform standard of service is developed and maintained even if the receptionist is absent from work.

The reception area

The reception area is the most important part of a salon because it is the focal point for all enquiries and information. The appearance of the reception is often the deciding factor in whether a client will make an appointment or not. An untidy reception occupied by a scruffy receptionist with unkempt hair, who is smoking and drinking coffee, does not promote an image that would attract clients. It is this part of the salon that deals with the greatest client traffic. Make the most of this opportunity by displaying promotion material and merchandise. Ideally, a reception area should provide the following:

- a comfortable waiting area;
- magazines, style books, product leaflets;
- refreshments;
- pleasant surroundings;
- sales point;
- retail displays and special promotions;
- a full list of salon services and prices;
- storage for clients' coats and salon gowns;
- information on whether a stylist is away or is running late.

2.3 The receptionist

Good reception skills are invaluable and people with them are worth their weight in gold. The first impression of the salon should be positive; both professional and caring. Clients expect all salon staff to be well turned out, from head to toe. Ideally, the receptionist should present an image of what the salon is trying to project. If a salon is known for short styles and the receptionist has long flowing locks, a false image of what should be expected is projected.

Appearances are not everything. The way the client is treated can also create the right impression. All clients should feel valued. Set out below are the fundamental dos and don'ts of how to deal with clients at the reception area:

Dos	*Don'ts*
Do be positive	Don't be curt or rude.
Do show friendliness and *smile*.	Don't act aloof or bored.
Do offer an alternative appointment at another time if you are fully booked.	Don't apologise and offer the client nothing instead of you are fully booked.
Do call the client by name.	Don't refer to 'Jane's 10.15', it sounds like a train!
Do apologise for any delay to an appointment.	Don't keep the client waiting without giving an explanation.
Do get up and show her where to sit.	Don't remain seated and wave her in the direction of where she should wait.
Do take the client's coat and help her put her gown on.	
Do speak clearly and look at the client, giving her your undivided attention.	Don't mumble or be more interested in what is going on around you.
Do excuse yourself if you need to answer the telephone during your conversation with the client.	Don't try to ignore the ringing of the phone while talking to the client.

Do ask the client if she would like tea, coffee, or magazines.

Don't leave it to the client to help herself or go without.

Never talk about a client if there is any possibility of being overheard by other clients; they will assume that what is said about one is said about others.

2.4 Telephone technique

The difference between speaking to someone on the telephone compared with a face to face situation, is that the other person is only *hearing* what you say. Because you cannot see the facial expressions or gestures, it is very easy to misinterpret what is being said. It is only the tone in the voice that conveys extra information about how a person feels. It is very easy to sound aggressive or be abrupt on the telephone. Remember, you will probably be dealing with some awkward clients over the telephone, but you are still expected to be helpful and polite. Here are some useful tips on telephone technique:

- Answer the telephone as quickly as possible, don't allow it to ring for ages as it creates a bad impression on the client who is phoning, as well as other clients in the salon. Avoid asking a client to hold if at all possible.
- Always hold the receiver of the phone a few inches from your mouth so that your voice is clearly picked up and heard. Never hold the receiver under your chin or you will sound quiet. Holding it too close to the mouth can muffle the voice. Also, never chew gum or eat while answering the phone.
- Always identify to the caller the salon's name when you answer the phone. Then say, 'Good morning, how can I help you?' Never just say 'Hello' when you answer the phone.
- Be polite and friendly. Speak clearly, using the clients' name, once you know who you are speaking to. Never mumble, shout, whisper, or be rude. Avoid the use of slang or being over-familiar to the caller, such as 'Hang on a sec., love!'.
- If ever you find it difficult to understand a client, blame the bad line and ask them to speak more slowly. Never tell callers that you are unable to understand their accent!
- Summarise the conversation to confirm what has been said, for example: 'Your appointment is at 3.15 pm next Friday, the 6th of the month'. This confirms what has been said for both you and the client. Include information such as the stylist and service required.
- Always end the call by thanking the client.

28 Cutting and Styling: a salon handbook

- Take a phone number or house number to confirm who the client was, in case you have two Mrs Mary Smiths.
- If you take a message on the telephone, do it properly. Use a message pad such as the one shown in Fig. 2.1. Take note of who the call was from, at what time it was taken, is there a message or a telephone number at which the person can be reached? Never rely on your memory or the fact that someone should know the telephone number of the person calling.

Fig. 2.1 A typical telephone message pad which can be used to take down messages which include relevant details.

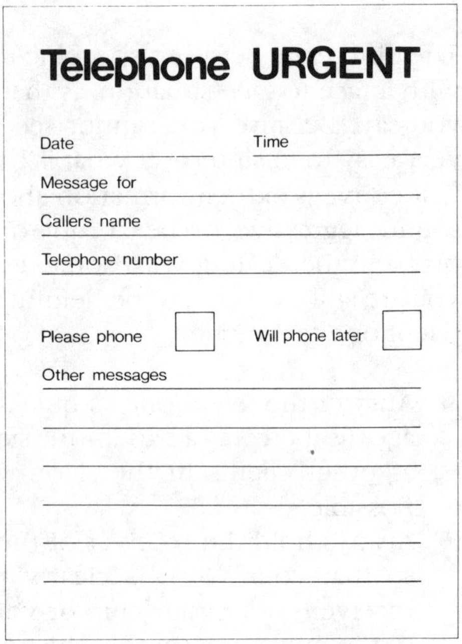

2.5 Making appointments

An appointment book is used to record all the appointments that clients make. Each appointment should be recorded in detail, noting the date, time, the client's name, the required service and the name of the stylist who will be attending to the client. The amount of time allocated for a specific service will vary from salon to salon, and also between faster and slower stylists. Likewise, the abbreviations used to describe a particular service will vary. For example, here are a few abbreviations used to describe particular services at one London salon:

S/S – shampoo and set
CBD – cut and blow dry
HL – highlights
PW – perm

Some salons also use codes to identify their clients:

* – new client
R – regular client
® – recommended client

Such codes can be used to calculate the number of new clients and regular clients over a specific period of time – especially useful, for instance, if the salon wants to assess the effectiveness of a recent advertising campaign. Usually, depending on salon size, a single sheet is used for each day. Such a sheet is shown in Fig. 2.2.

DATE: Monday 18th March			
	Steve	Jane	Pauline
8.30 a.m.			
8.45			
9.0	A. Wilson®	Mrs Day s/s	Christine
9.15	CBD	Mrs Cane®	CBD
9.30	P. Briant*	PW	Mr Shaw R
9.45	C s/s	//////	CBD
10.0	Mrs Shaw*	F. Wilson*	P. Andrews*
10.15	HL (Long Hair)	CBD	CBD
10.30	//////	M. Elson*	Mrs Starr s/s
10.45	\\\\\\	C s/s	Mrs Mill c s/s ®
11.0	Mrs May ®		//////
11.15	CBD		
11.30	F. Timms^R s/s	Mrs Penfold BD	Mrs March *
11.45			Tint

Fig. 2.2 A page taken from an appointments book showing the columns of three stylists.

Alternatively, the salon may use a computer to record the appointments, in which case a special program may need to be bought or written for the salon to accommodate the necessary information.

Once the appointment has been made for a client at reception, write down the date, time and stylist for the client on their appointment card. If you do this, there is no chance of a misunderstanding, so do it clearly!

Making appointments — some points to remember:

- Write in pencil in the appointment book so that it can be erased if an appointment should be cancelled.

- Write clearly so that it can be read by anyone who may need to look at the appointment book.
- Concentrate to avoid making mistakes.
- If an appointment is cancelled, immediately erase the client's name so that the space can be filled.
- Allocate the correct amount of time for each service. Perms will take longer to carry out than blow dries.
- Record each appointment in full detail.
- When a client makes an appointment, stress that an early notification of a cancellation would be appreciated so that another client can be placed.

Another important part of the receptionist's job is to handle cash transactions. This is dealt with fully in Chapter 9 – *Salon Organisation*.

2.6 Non-verbal communication

Hairdressing is an occupation which revolves around a skill which is probably the most important of all the qualities that a hairdresser needs to possess. This all important skill is the ability to communicate effectively with those we work alongside and, of course, our clients.

Hairdressers need to be good communicators, patient listeners, always cheerful, pleasant, polite, and of course, excellent at their work. It seems a lot to ask of anybody, especially on the morning you go to work feeling under the weather with a busy day ahead of you. It takes a great deal of effort to smile and cheerfully welcome the client that you dread coming to the salon, but the professional hairdresser will always treat all clients equally, no matter how they feel towards individuals.

Being aware of how to 'read' the non-verbal communication or language of others can help us to understand certain situations more fully and how best to deal with them. For example, a client storming through the salon door, with her jaw jutting forward, eyes narrowed and fists clenched is obviously an angry person! When we meet an aggressive situation such as this, an equally aggressive approach would do very little to promote good human relationships. The recognition of non-verbal communication affects the ways in which we respond to others, and also the ways in which others respond to us. Non-verbal communication can be broken down into the following areas:

- posture and stance
- gestures
- facial expressions

- eye contact
- clothes, jewellery and other accessories.

Posture and stance

The ways in which people 'arrange their bodies' as they stand or sit may be extremely communicative. As a general rule, the body frame is more widely spread in a relaxed position, whether seated or standing, when someone feels at ease. If, however, a person is experiencing discomfort, nervousness or tension, the body is more tightly held, with arms and legs together, occupying less space.

The ability to interpret such signals and to act as necessary, to disarm or reassure, is invaluable in promoting good relations. If a client is uptight after being kept waiting, it is important to recognise this and compensate for it in your actions and attitude towards them. What messages do the stick men communicate in the examples shown in Fig. 2.3?

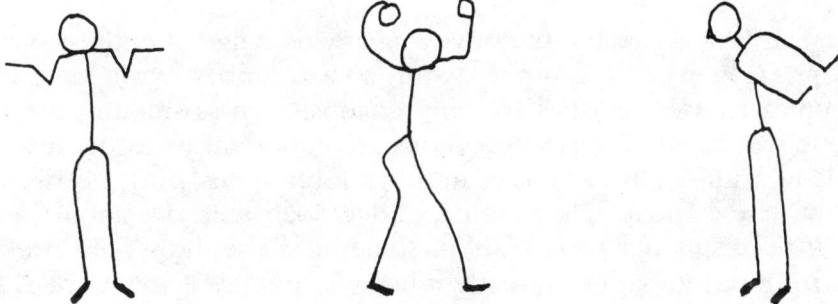

Fig. 2.3 Examples of postures which show certain attitudes.

Gestures

When people communicate, they do so both verbally and non-verbally. As they speak they move their hands, head and body. These movements are closely co-ordinated with their speech, and form part of the total communication.

Some gestures are consciously and deliberately made. For, example, the car driver who points his finger to his head with a screwing motion is demonstrating what he thinks about the quality of someone's driving! We use gestures to give illustrations of size, shape and movement. This is particularly useful in hairdressing when something is difficult to describe in words.

When people are emotionally aroused, they produce apparently pointless body movements that reflect their emotional state. People often touch themselves when experiencing certain emotions. Examples include:

- fist clenching – aggression
- face touching – anxiety
- scratching – self-blame
- forehead wiping – tiredness.

Head-nods are a rather special kind of gesture, and have a distinctive role. They act as reinforcers; that is, they reward and encourage what has gone before. They can also be used to encourage someone to talk more. A nod usually means that the speaker should carry on, but a rapid succession of nods may mean that the listener would like to speak himself. Tilting the head to one side and holding eye contact tells the other person that you are listening to what he or she is saying.

Facial expression

The human face is capable of conveying a wide range of expressions and emotions. However, it is under your control and so can be used to communicate false messages and impressions, such as smiling sweetly at someone we dislike. Facial expressions are important to us because they provide us with feedback. For example, if John smiles, nods his head and agrees whenever Joan talks about politics, Joan will talk about politics more. If he wants her to talk about something else, he would probably frown and not look at her directly whenever politics is mentioned. Here are a few examples of facial expression:

- Eyebrows: fully raised – disbelief
  half raised – surprise
  half lowered – puzzled
  fully lowered – angry, disapproving
- Mouth: up-turned – pleasure
  down-turned – displeasure

Eye contact

Eyes are an important means of feedback. They can express friendliness or hostility, and people regard them as an important communicator of character. We have all heard the expression that someone 'has shifty eyes'. If you feel this to be true about someone you will not trust him.

Basically, if we hold eye contact with someone, it tells them that we are interested in them or what they are saying. This can be used to show general interest, love, lust, anger or sympathy. Gazing upwards expresses disinterest and total avoidance of eye contact can show disinterest, dislike, dissatisfaction or shyness.

If a client avoids eye contact with herself in the mirror while you are doing her hair, it could mean that she does not like what you are doing with her hair!

Clothes, jewellery and other accessories

Our appearance is the initial way in which we promote ourselves to others. The expression that someone 'looks loaded' can only be made on the surface, as we cannot see their bank balance! People who are aware that they are projecting a favourable image (by means of positive feedback) not only feel better for it, but also have more self-confidence and self-assurance.

We judge others by the way they look and come to certain conclusions about the person, even though we may not have had contact with them. All of us do this, subconsciously, all the time. Think about when a new client enters the salon. The moment you look at her, you are bombarded with information in the form of the non-verbal signals that we have already touched upon. The clothes that a person wears will tell you a lot. You will come to definite conclusions about lifestyle, financial position, character and age very quickly, based purely on looks. Jewellery and other accessories such as sunglasses, silk scarves, etc., will also give you clues about whom you are dealing with.

If you are aiming to support and reinforce this image by the service you are offering, you must be able to interpret these signals. The final service you offer should be determined by a sequence of both verbal and non-verbal communication.

This human communication process is extremely complex, but every hairdresser should be aware of how important it is to promote meaningful communication within the salon.

2.7 Persuasive communication

Stylists will often miss golden opportunities of persuading a client to have a particular service or buying a specific product. Why does this happen? Perhaps the best way of analysing this situation is to understand a little of the psychology of selling.

Imagine that a client has made an appointment with you for a cut and blow dry. While looking at her hair and discussing what she wants, your judgement tells you that her hair would benefit from having a special treatment because it is out of condition. We can look at that example in the form of the diagram shown in Fig. 2.4.

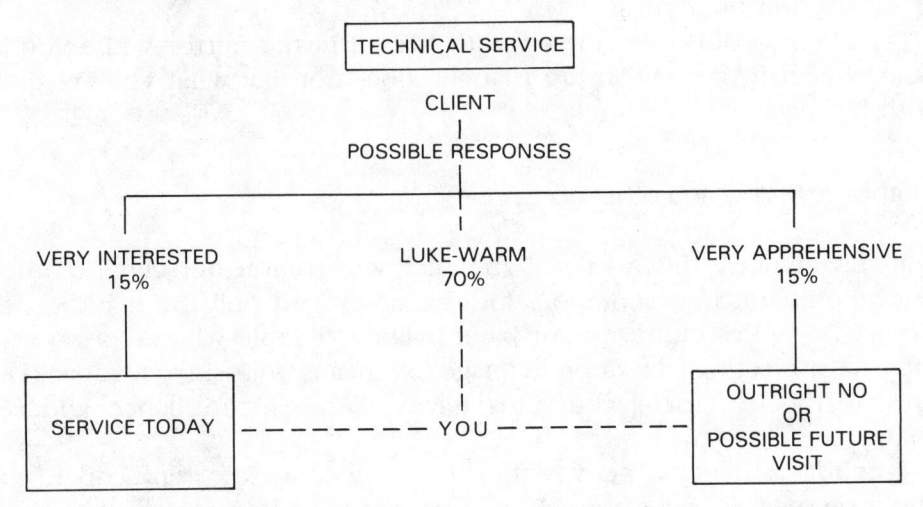

```
                    TECHNICAL SERVICE
                          CLIENT
                    POSSIBLE RESPONSES

    VERY INTERESTED      LUKE-WARM       VERY APPREHENSIVE
         15%                70%                 15%

                                              OUTRIGHT NO
                                                  OR
      SERVICE TODAY  — — — — YOU — — — —   POSSIBLE FUTURE
                                                 VISIT
```

Fig. 2.4 The possible responses of a client to extra service. (Courtesy of L'Oréal.)

As you can see from the diagram, the majority of clients fall into the 'lukewarm' category, and it is your influence on such clients which could be defined as selling. However, never push a client into a service she neither wants, needs nor can afford – this is bad selling and is ultimately bad for business. Clients must always feel at ease, or they will not return. If it is a good product that will benefit their hair and appearance, they will appreciate your interest. The process of selling can be divided into three steps:

(1) analysing the client's needs;
(2) giving advice (introducing the service or product);
(3) gaining agreement on how to meet these needs, if required.

Let us look at these three steps in more detail.

Step (1). Analysing the client's needs can be done by:

- Establishing a relationship by developing interest and trust.
- Asking questions which begin with How? When? Where? Why? and Which?
- Demonstrating understanding by using visual aids such as style books or product leaflets.
- Formulating an opinion which will rely on your technical knowledge.

Step (2). Giving advice is done by:

- Explaining the service in terms of what it will do for the client.
- Convincing the client of these benefits.
- Being enthusiastic and having a positive belief in the service that you are recommending.

Step (3). Gaining agreement is achieved when your client is interested by:

- Suggesting that the service is given at that moment.
- Reassuring the client if she is still apprehensive and perhaps suggesting more modest alternatives.

2.8 Salon retailing

It is true to say that most clients buy their shampoo, hair spray, mousse, and conditioners from supermarkets with the weekly shopping, or from the chemist. Why? Because salons are not promoted as the places where they should buy them. Millions of pounds worth of haircare products are being sold through a vast number of retail outlets. Currently this is a £400 million a year market. If salons could take just 5 per cent of this market it would generate an extra £20 million of turnover each year! Just an extra £25 worth of retail profit per week generates over £1000 additional profit a year.

Here are some quotes from those who really know about retailing:

'Selling should be included in every normal training programme.' (*Wella*)

'With more and more clients visiting the salon less and less often, the only growth area in salon business is through retailing.' (*Redken*)

'Recommendation from a professional is something you don't get at the local chemist.' (*Schwarzkopf*)

'We are getting daily phone calls from people whose total business has trebled.' (*L'Oréal*)

Research shows that clients want more advice from their hairdressers about what products they should be using on their hair. Usually, they do not get it. To be professional, stylists need to analyse clients' needs and give them good advice. As a stylist, you have the undivided attention of your client during each appointment, but do you take advantage of it?

How much better it would make your service if you spent time talking to the client about what she thinks of her hair and what products she uses at home. A careful lowering of the eyebrows will have the client asking you what you would recommend. Sadly, a client will usually learn more about haircare from women's magazines and television commercials than from the person who knows her hair personally – her hairdresser.

Salon retailing can be a very profitable business. Not only is your standard of service improved by analysing your client's needs and recommending the appropriate home products but you may also draw prospective clients into your salon through an attractive product display. Another advantage of retailing is giving the client a bag bearing the salon name to take the products home in. It is an advertisement wherever it is carried. These are some simple guidelines for displaying goods in the salon:

Dos	*Don'ts*
Do display all of your stock as a large amount attracts more interest.	Don't leave most of your stock in the stockroom where it can't be seen.
Do mark every product clearly with its price.	Don't leave products unpriced; clients may be reluctant to ask you the price.
Do make sure that the goods are easy to see and accessible.	Don't have goods under lock and key as clients will be reluctant to ask you to take them out.
Do make displays large to attract attention.	Don't set up too many small displays as they have less impact.
Do use your salon window and entrance area to let passers-by know that you sell retail goods.	Don't miss the opportunity to exploit your salon frontage to its full extent.
Do make displays attractive and change them regularly.	Don't leave items in the window until they are faded, or use damaged items.

It is vitally important to get your staff interested in selling products. This can be done in a variety of ways, including commission, profit-sharing for the whole salon, and simply using the products in the salon.

2.9 Questions

1. Why is it important to be able to communicate well with your clients?
2. What will a client expect from a visit to the salon?
3. Why is the reception area so important to a salon?
4. What points would you consider when designing a reception area for a salon?
5. Why is it important for salon prices to be fully displayed?
6. How can a receptionist reflect the image of a salon?
7. List what you would consider as the five most important do's and don'ts for a receptionist.
8. What differences are there between talking to a client in person or on the telephone?
9. What would you do if you could not understand a client on the telephone?
10. When you answer the phone, what is the first thing that you should say?
11. Why should you summarise a conversation at the end of a telephone call?
12. If you take a message on the telephone, what kinds of things should it detail and why?
13. Why are letters used as a shorthand for services in an appointments book?
14. Why might it be helpful to know if clients are regular, new or recommended?
15. Why should an appointment be written in pencil?
16. What advantage is there for the salon if you write down the client's appointment on their card?
17. What is non-verbal communication?
18. How can this be broken down into different areas?
19. How can posture and stance tell you how a person feels?
20. How can gestures tell you how a person feels?
21. Describe how the eyebrows can show different feelings.
22. Describe how the movement of the mouth can show different feelings.
23. Why is it good to make eye contact with someone?
24. What can clothes and jewellery tell you about a client?
25. What percentage of clients are usually not interested at all in any other service?
26. How would you go about trying to interest a client in an extra service on a salon visit?
27. Why is it a bad thing to pursue a retail sale if the client is not interested?

38　Cutting and Styling: a salon handbook

28　Why is salon retailing a possible growth area for salons?
29　What do you consider the five most important things about a salon retail display?
30　What types of things do you think that your salon could sell that it does not already?
31　If you owned a salon, how would you get the interest of staff aroused in retail selling?

3
Equipment and Tools

Do you remember your first day in the salon? Wondering what all the equipment surrounding you was used for? It can be confusing, learning what each item is called, and how and when you use it. This chapter aims to tell you about the types of equipment and tools you are likely to come across while working in the salon, emphasising safe handling and maintenance. The chapter will deal with equipment in four broad areas:

- salon fittings and equipment;
- electrical appliances;
- hairdressing tools;
- haircutting tools.

3.1 Salon fittings and equipment

Basins

The backwash type of basin shown in Fig. 3.1 is the type most often seen in salons today, although forward shampoo basins were once very popular. The forward type required the client to sit over the basin to have a shampoo. Its decline in popularity came about when the backwash basin, which has the advantages of increased client comfort and safety, was designed. Using the backwash basin makes it far easier to ensure that chemicals do not enter clients' eyes. With the forward wash, on the other hand, even towels held against the face did not stop the face from getting wet.

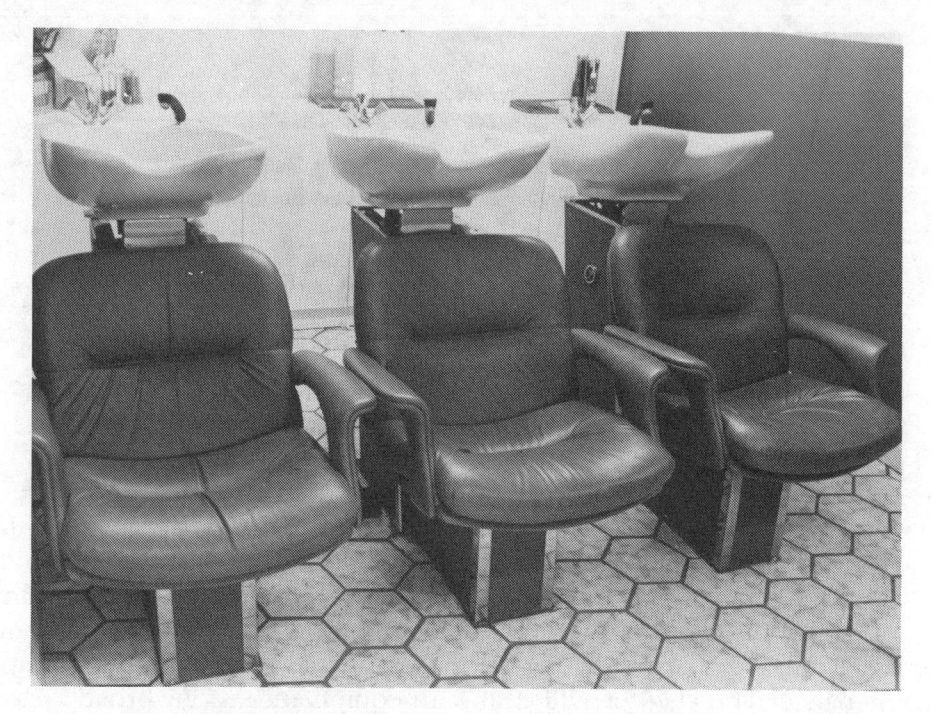

Fig. 3.1 Backwash basins installed as an island unit, complete with chairs. The mixer taps enable the correct water temperature to be selected. (Courtesy of Pietranera (UK) Ltd.)

The backwash basin requires the client to recline so that the neck rests in the hollow at the front of the basin. It is extremely important that the correct height of chair is used, otherwise it can be very uncomfortable for the client if this factor has not been given adequate consideration in the initial planning of the salon. Backwashes may be bought either as a complete unit, consisting of a housing unit, mixer taps, spray and chair, or can be obtained individually. As models vary so much, the salon owner can choose between a wide range of colours and styles. They can be installed either as an island fitment, so that the operator can choose between standing at the side or behind the client, or can be plumbed in against a wall, so that the stylist can only shampoo hair from the side.

Mixer taps enable the operator to adjust the water temperature accurately. The cold water should always be turned on first, adding hot water until the correct temperature is reached. This prevents the risk of scalding the client (or yourself!), as well as preserving the life of the hose. The spray should not be too heavy, or it may crack the basin if it is dropped. Although hoses and sprays vary, it is the water pressure of the salon that finally dictates how forceful the force of water can be.

Equipment and Tools 41

Underneath the basin there will be a U-bend or bottle trap, whose purpose is to prevent odours or air-borne infections coming up from the drains. However, as clients lose hairs (quite naturally) when their hair is shampooed, the trap may become blocked with hair. This becomes noticeable when water does not flow away freely. Always check to see if the trap is blocked before taking the expensive step of calling in the plumber. It is a simple, although slightly unpleasant, procedure to clean it. The two types of trap are illustrated in Fig. 3.2.

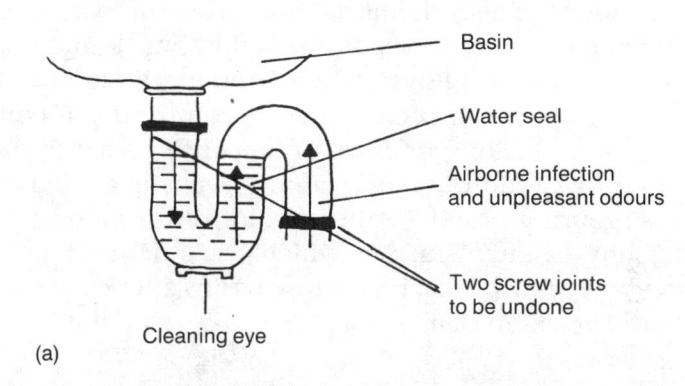

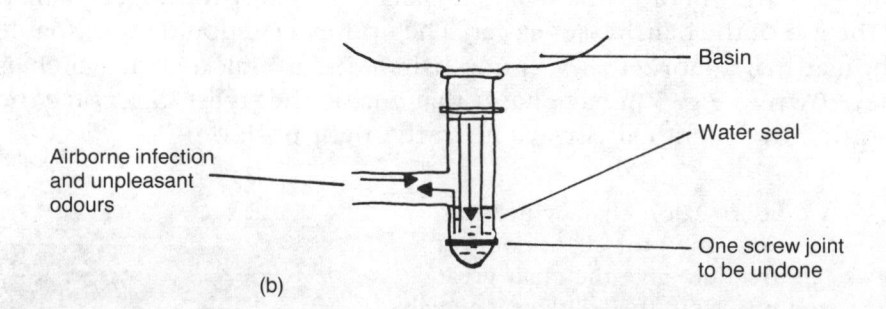

Fig. 3.2 (a) U-bend and (b) a bottle trap under a shampoo basin. Note that the U-bend is actually an S-trap, as can be seen from its shape.

Unblocking a trap

(1) Place a bucket underneath the trap.
(2) Unscrew the trap sealing ring(s) and let the water and blockage fall into the bucket. A small piece of wire may help you remove the hair.
(3) Replace the trap and tighten the sealing ring(s).
   Let some water run to seal the trap again, checking underneath that you have sealed it properly and that there are no leaks.

(4) Dispose of the contents of the bucket down the toilet.

If there should be an accident in the salon and either a piece of jewellery or a contact lens falls down the sink plughole, turn off the water immediately. Contacts will often float for a while. If you open the trap, as has just been described, there is a good chance that the lost item will still be in the trap.

Alternatively, blocked drains (traps and gulleys) can be cleared by using caustic soda. This chemical must be prepared according to the manufacturer's instructions, as it is highly caustic and can cause severe skin burns. Wear rubber gloves when handling it and wash off any spillages with plenty of running cold water. If you try this it could save you many pounds as unblocking drains is an expensive service.

A note of caution about cleaning basins. Never use abrasive cleaners such as scouring powders; these will take the shine off the porcelain and create tiny scratch marks which can harbour germs and become progressively more unsightly. Rinse basins after each client so that they are not left covered in hair or soap suds.

Chairs

Because clients have to sit in salon chairs for long periods of time, comfort is very important. A comfortable client is also less likely to 'fidget', which makes the job of the hairdresser easier. The upholstery should be washable and not made of a fabric that will trap hairs. Modern salon chairs, such as the one shown in Fig. 3.3, have bases that enable the stylist to revolve the chair so that the client can always be in the right position.

Fig. 3.3 A modern salon chair which has been designed for client comfort. The five feet give the chair great stability. Note the solid arms which will wear better than cloth-upholstered ones. (Courtesy of Pietranera (UK) Ltd.)

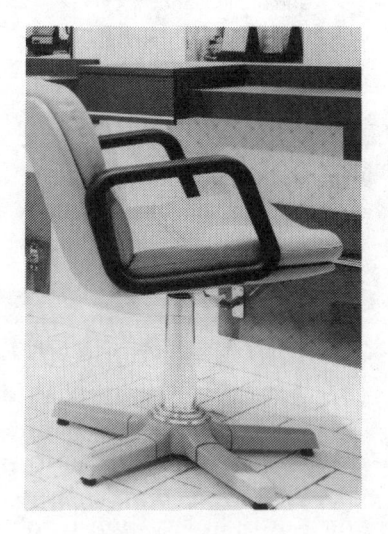

Some chairs are hydraulic or semi-hydraulic; this means that the height of the seat can be adjusted by either pulling a lever or pressing a pump with the foot. Obviously it makes a stylist's job a lot easier if the chairs are adjustable because it saves excessive bending, which can cause backache and fatigue. Chairs can have many different features including neckrests, footrests and reclining backrests. A word of warning: if your styling units have sharp edges which chairs can be pushed against or under, avoid padded arms rests. They can tear within weeks, so choose solid moulded plastic or metal instead.

Chairs should be wiped or brushed down after they have been used for a haircut so that the next client is not presented with a hair-covered seat. At least once a week, all salon chairs should be washed down and any metal parts polished. Special plastic covers are available to slip over the back of chairs to protect them from staining. If tint does accidentally drip onto a chair, wipe it off immediately to prevent staining.

3.2 Electrical appliances

All electrical appliances that are used in a salon should have a British Standards number to show that they meet minimum safety requirements. Never use an appliance with wet hands, nor if it has a cracked plug or damaged cable. *If there is an accident it is the salon owner who will be prosecuted.* If an appliance needs servicing, always disconnect from the mains and always consult an electrician if in doubt. Electricity can kill, so treat it with respect. If used properly, electric tools make the life of the hairdresser much easier.

About 200 deaths result each year as a result of electrical accidents. Obey safety rules!

Hairdriers (hand-held)

A professional hand-held drier has a much longer lifespan than an ordinary consumer model, enabling it to withstand constant daily use in salons. An example of a professional hairdrier is shown in Fig. 3.4. They should be lightweight, well-balanced, and have variable heat and speed controls. This enables the stylist to adjust air temperature and flow rate according to the type of hair being styled.

The flex should be long enough to enable the stylist to work easily on all sides of the head, without draping it over the client! To prevent the flex from becoming damaged the drier can be hung up on its built-in hook, so that the flex does not become twisted. When storing the drier in a bag or cupboard, always wrap the flex in a figure of eight around the handle and

44 Cutting and Styling: a salon handbook

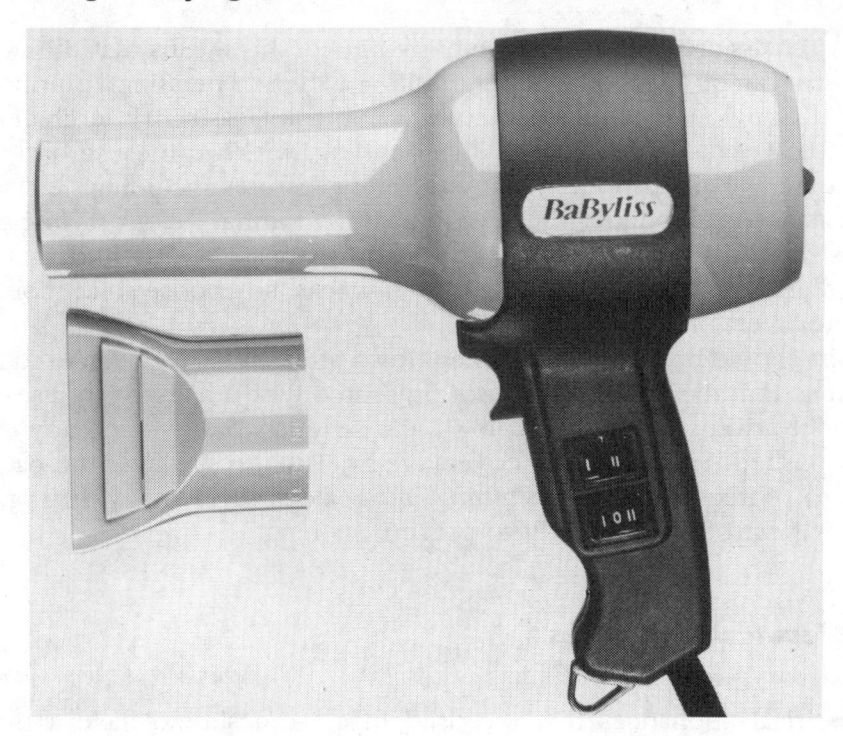

Fig. 3.4 A professional hairdrier complete with nozzle. Controls for variable air flow speed and temperature are incorporated into the handle. (Courtesy of Babyliss Ltd.)

neck of the drier. This prevents pull on the wires inside the drier and stops the flex from becoming damaged. If the flex is wound tightly around the handle, the wires inside the flex may become brittle and fracture, causing electric shorting out. The flex will also have a tendency to coil up while you are working.

The back of these types of drier have a filter which prevents dust particles from entering the motor inside. This will require regular cleaning as a build-up of dust reduces the amount of cool air that the hairdrier can suck in, causing it to overheat and cut out. This is a safety mechanism to prevent the hairdrier from serious overheating and possibly catching fire. Disconnect the hairdrier from its socket before you clean the filter, and never work without this filter being in place, as hair could be sucked up into the fan. For this reason, a stylist with long hair should wear it tied back.

Hairdriers can be used with or without the nozzle as all this does is change the concentration of the airflow. When a nozzle is used the airflow is forced through a narrow slit which concentrates its force (see Fig. 3.5(b)). Without a nozzle the airflow leaves the drier at a much wider angle (see Fig. 3.5(a)).

Equipment and Tools

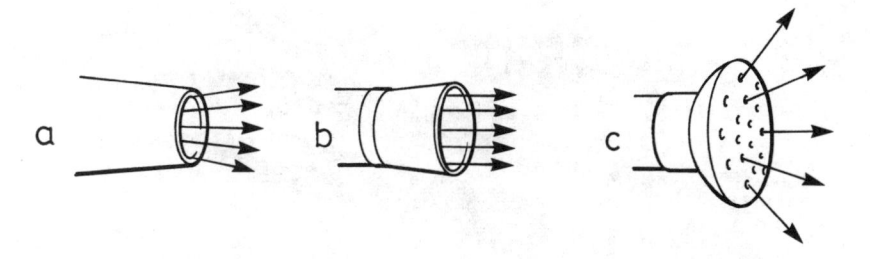

Fig. 3.5 The varying airflow of hairdriers: (a) without a nozzle; (b) with a nozzle; and (c) with a diffuser attachment.

Special attachments, called diffusers, can be bought to attach to a drier. These disperse the air at a very wide angle and are particularly useful if a style needs minimal disturbance from the airflow (see Fig. 3.5(c)).

Safe working guide — hairdriers

- Always work with a clean filter in place.
- Never use a hairdrier if the plug is cracked or the flex is damaged.
- Never use a hairdrier with wet hands.
- Never leave cables where people could trip over them.
- Always switch a hairdrier off before putting it down. The vibration of the motor could cause it to move and fall to the ground.
- Never hold a hairdrier too close to a client's scalp. It can burn the skin and scorch the hair. For the same reason, do not play a stream of hot air on one area too long, especially if the hair has metal clips that might heat up. If you doubt this, try holding your hand near the airflow when your drier is on hot!
- For an explanation of the physical changes in hair when blow drying or using tongs, please see Chapter 6.

Hot brushes

Hot brushes have become increasingly popular in both the professional trade and the home consumer market. Many people find them easier to handle than tongs because the hair tends to cling to the teeth. The hot brushes shown in Fig. 3.6 are available in three different sizes for creating different sized curls. All hot brushes are fitted with a thermostatic control which prevents overheating. However, leaving them on all day will undoubtedly affect the lifespan of such an appliance.

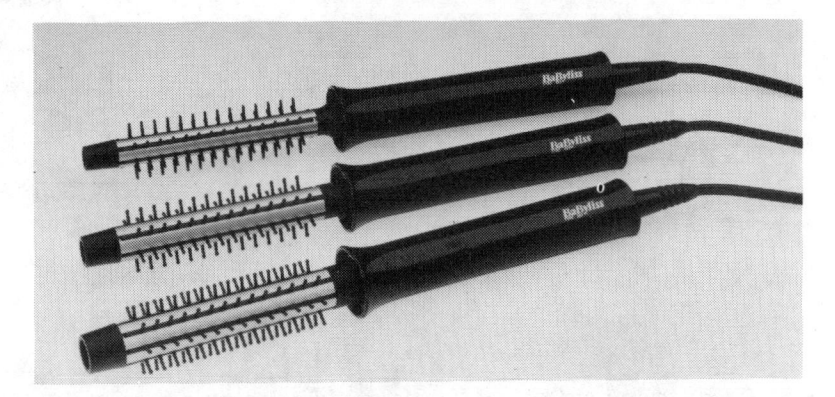

Fig. 3.6 A selection of different sized hot brushes. (Courtesy of Babyliss Ltd.)

The flex of a hot brush has a swivel action so that during the turning of the brush, the flex does not twist or tangle. The points of the hair must be cleanly wrapped around the brush to prevent buckled and distorted ends. The hot brush is wound down so that the entire length of the hair is wrapped around it. Placing a comb between the hot brush and the scalp will ensure that the heat does not cause discomfort to the client. The hot brush is held in the hair for several seconds until the heat has penetrated through the mesh of hair (you can test that this has happened with your fingers). When the hair has been heated sufficiently, the hot brush is gently removed by carefully unwinding it. The hair should be allowed to cool thoroughly before it is combed or brushed.

There are hot brushes available without cords which are described as 'independent'. They use butane cartridges or batteries to provide the energy to produce heat. They are popular to take on holidays, or for hairdressers who are involved in photographic location work.

Safe working guide — hot brushes

- Do not leave hot brushes switched on longer than necessary, as this will shorten their working life and make it more likely for accidents to occur.
- Clean them regularly with the power disconnected. Use some cotton wool dampened with methylated spirit to remove dirt. Never immerse in water to clean.
- Take clean sections so that the brush does not get tangled in the hair.
- Because damaged hair cannot withstand as much heat as hair in good condition, make allowances when using the hot brush.
- Wait until the hot brush has cooled before putting it away into a bag or cupboard.

Tongs

Tongs, otherwise known as curling irons, are used to curl hair and differ from hot brushes because there is a smooth surface on the curling rod. The example shown in Fig. 3.7 has a built-in stand which can be used for resting the tongs when they are not being used. The black tip at the end of the metal rod is a safety tip which enables the stylist to hold the tongs for extra control.

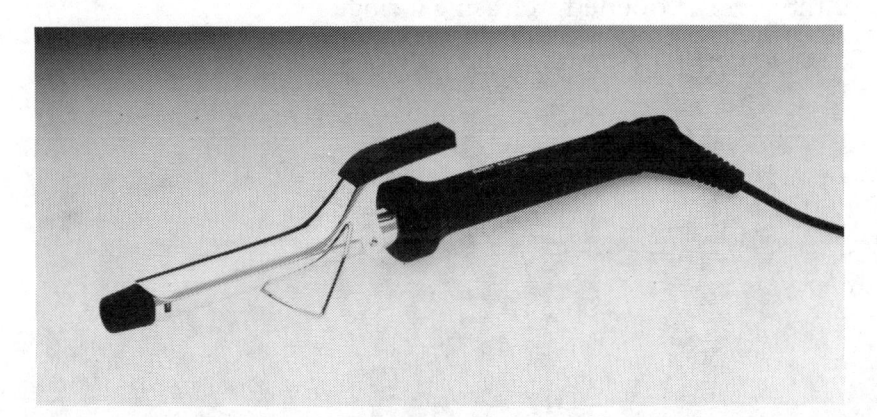

Fig. 3.7 Modern electric curling tongs shown resting on their stand. (Courtesy of Babyliss Ltd.)

The flex has a swivel action to prevent the cord from tangling, allowing easier manipulation. The lever opens the tongs as it is depressed, then it is closed on the mesh of hair once the points are cleanly wrapped around the rod. The tongs are wound up the hair length and held in position until the heat has penetrated through the hair mesh. If curling right up to the roots, place a vulcanite comb between the tongs and the scalp to act as a barrier against the heat, as shown in Fig. 3.8. Once the hair is released from the tongs, it should be allowed to cool before it is combed or brushed.

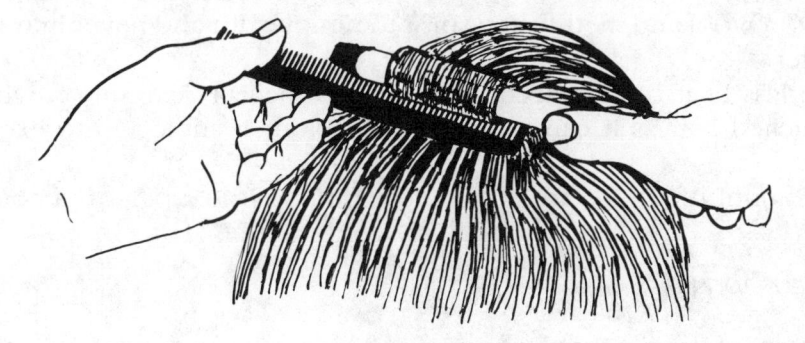

Fig. 3.8 Protecting the scalp while using curling tongs. A heat-resistant comb is inserted between the scalp and the tongs.

Spiral tongs

Spiral tongs are curling irons which have a spiral groove running down the heated rod. Figure 3.9 shows a modern electric pair. This type of tongs has the same features as the ordinary tongs; built-in rest, protective safety tip and swivel flex. The lever is depressed and is closed on the hair points. As the tongs are turned, the mesh of hair will automatically position itself in the spiral groove running down the rod. Once the hair is sufficiently heated, the lever is opened, releasing a ringlet curl.

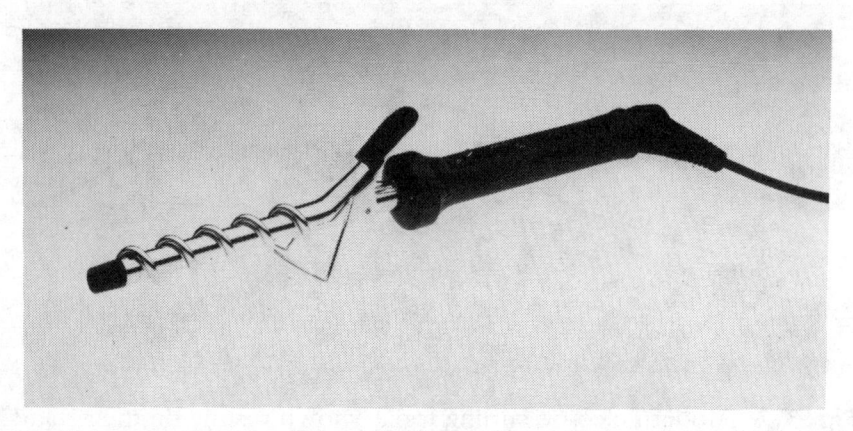

Fig. 3.9 Electric spiral tongs shown resting on their stand. (Courtesy of Babyliss Ltd.)

Safe working guide — tongs

- Do not leave the tongs switched on for longer than necessary as this will shorten the life of the appliance and increases the chance of accidents.
- Use the built-in stand to prevent the scorching of work surfaces.
- Clean the appliance regularly, while disconnected from the mains. Use cotton wool and methylated spirit to remove dirt and never immerse in water.
- Use less heat on damaged hair and be especially careful on white or bleached hair as it can noticeably discolour if subjected to excessive heat.
- Wait until the tongs are cool before putting into a bag or cupboard.

New wave tongs

These tongs consist of three styling rods and a movable plate as shown in Fig. 3.10, the third styling rod being under the plate. They are designed for creating deep, natural looking waves. This type of tongs has similar features to those already described, as they have a built-in rest and swivel flex. As the handle is depressed, the rods are closed against the grooves of the plate. If a slightly 'harder' effect is desired, rather like that from a marcel waving iron, remove the plate. The same safe working guide applies as for tongs.

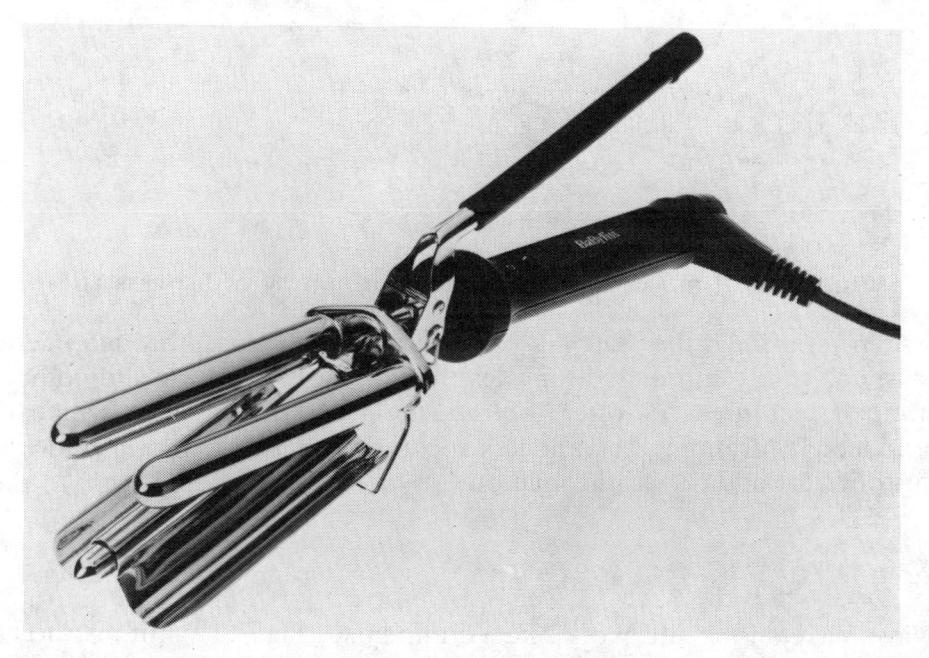

Fig. 3.10 The Babyliss New Wave can be used to create deep, natural looking waves. (Courtesy of Babyliss Ltd.)

Crimpers

Crimpers create straight line crimps in the hair in a uniform pattern. They can be used on all of the hair or in specific areas only, to produce a variety of effects. Crimpers, such as those shown in Fig. 3.11, can be used to produce an interesting texture for straight hair. They can increase its volume, making it appear thicker.

A mesh of hair is taken about 2 cms (1 inch) deep and no wider than the metal plates of the crimper. They are then carefully positioned so that the plates are on both sides of the hair mesh where the crimp effect is desired. The crimpers are closed and held in position for 2–5 seconds, depending on the quality of hair, and then released. This procedure can be carried out repeatedly down the length of the hair until all the hair is crimped. Crimping the underneath hair of bobs gives added fullness and support to lank hair.

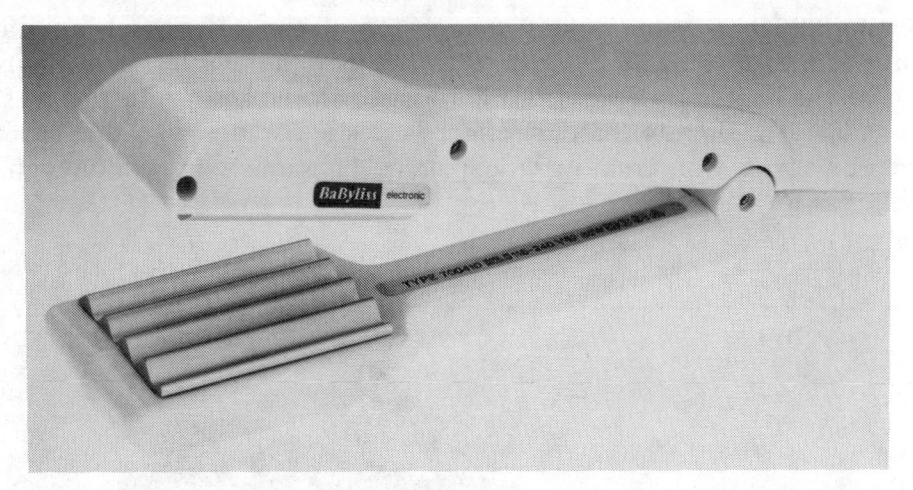

Fig. 3.11 A modern electric crimper. (Courtesy of Babyliss Ltd.)

After crimping the hair, it can either be combed through, gently brushed, or left untouched for a less natural look. Brushing and combing crimped hair gives a softer look as the hard zig-zag lines which are produced by crimping become less apparent. (See safe working guidelines for tongs for additional information.)

Wave makers

Wave Makers look and work like a crimper (see Fig. 3.12) but instead of a tight crimping effect, they create deeper, softer waves. They can be used all over, or on certain areas only. The hair can be gently combed with a wide-toothed comb or the fingers afterwards, or alternatively, can be left to give deep firm waves.

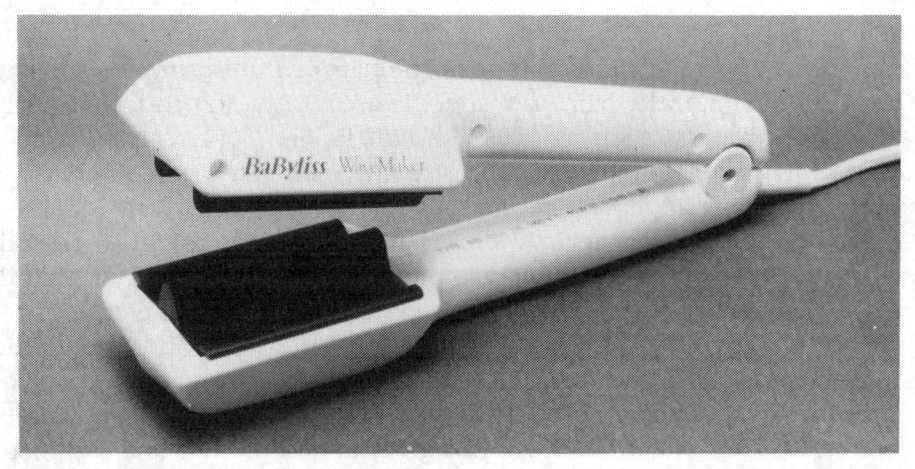

Fig. 3.12 An electric Wave Maker. (Courtesy of Babyliss Ltd.)

Straighteners

With most electrical hair appliances geared to curling or waving hair, it is refreshing to include straighteners. A modern electric straightener is illustrated in Fig. 3.13. It works on the same principle as the crimpers but instead of creating crimps or waves, it irons out the curl or frizz. Electric straighteners are particularly useful for pressing super-curly hair to produce straighter looks. Please see safe working guidelines for additional information.

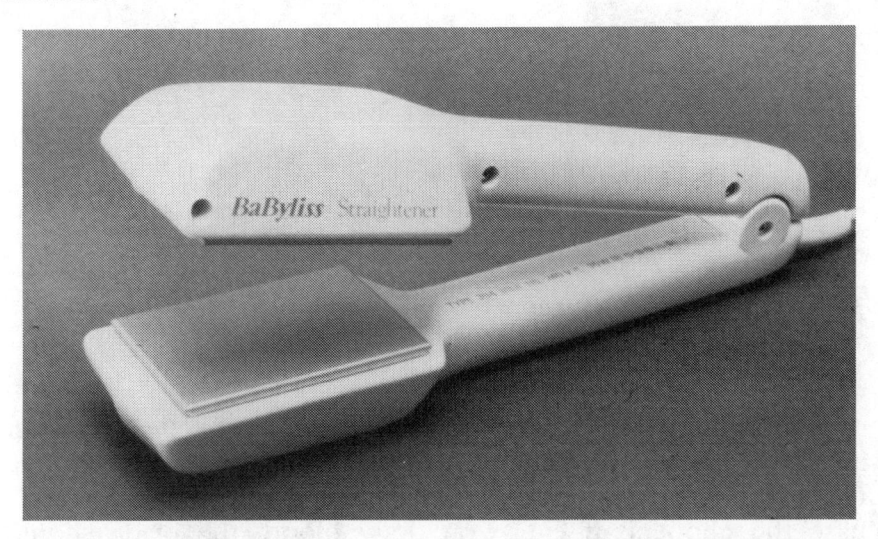

Fig. 3.13 An electric pair of straightening irons, the Straightener. (Courtesy of Babyliss Ltd.)

Electric clippers

Electric clippers have become increasingly popular in recent years for creating sharp and pronounced shapes on both European and black hair. They can be used to create strong outside shapes on the hairline only, or can be used to carry out a complete haircut.

Many types of electric clippers exist on the market, varying in weight, size and cutting precision. Rechargeable clippers are now available, meaning that they are totally portable, with an operating time of about 30 minutes before recharging is necessary. They are simply placed back into their special holding unit for recharging. The clippers shown in Fig. 3.14 can have the blades adjusted so that an exact amount of hair is removed.

Electric clippers work on the principle of one blade remaining fixed while the other moves across it. The action of the moving blade, operated by the motor, is similar to several pairs of scissors being used at the same time; as many as 14,400 cutting strokes can be made per minute with some types of clippers.

Basically, clippers are used by carefully placing in position and directing them as required. They are a particularly useful tool for creating etched lines in short styles and for cutting out partings in Afro hair.

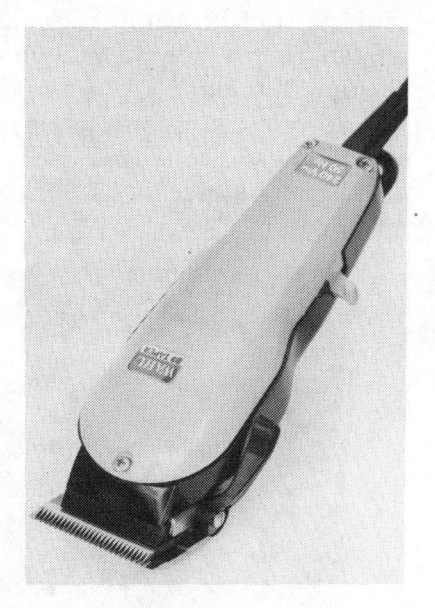

Fig. 3.14 A pair of electric clippers. (Courtesy of Wahl Ltd.)

It is important to keep your clipper blades well oiled with an oil specifically designed for that purpose. The blades should be aligned according to the manufacturer's instructions, so keep these when you purchase the clippers. If ever you draw blood, the blade should be removed and soaked in disinfectant, refitted, and finally re-oiled. Hopefully, one day, a manufacturer will come up with some clippers which are easier to take apart and reassemble.

Heated rollers

Heated rollers are an asset for many clients because they achieve quick results and are relatively easy for an unskilled person to use. However, they can also be useful in the salon for a quick set or for adding curl and bounce. They are invaluable for session work when the stylist needs to be quick and the model is shared with the make-up artist.

Figure 3.15 shows a set of heated rollers. There are different sized rollers and each is positioned over a metal bar which heats it up. On top of each roller is a red dot which turns black when fully heated, indicating that the rollers are ready for use. The machine takes about ten minutes to heat up the rollers, so this time should be allowed for if you are using them. Once heated the rollers are taken off their individual heating elements as they are needed.

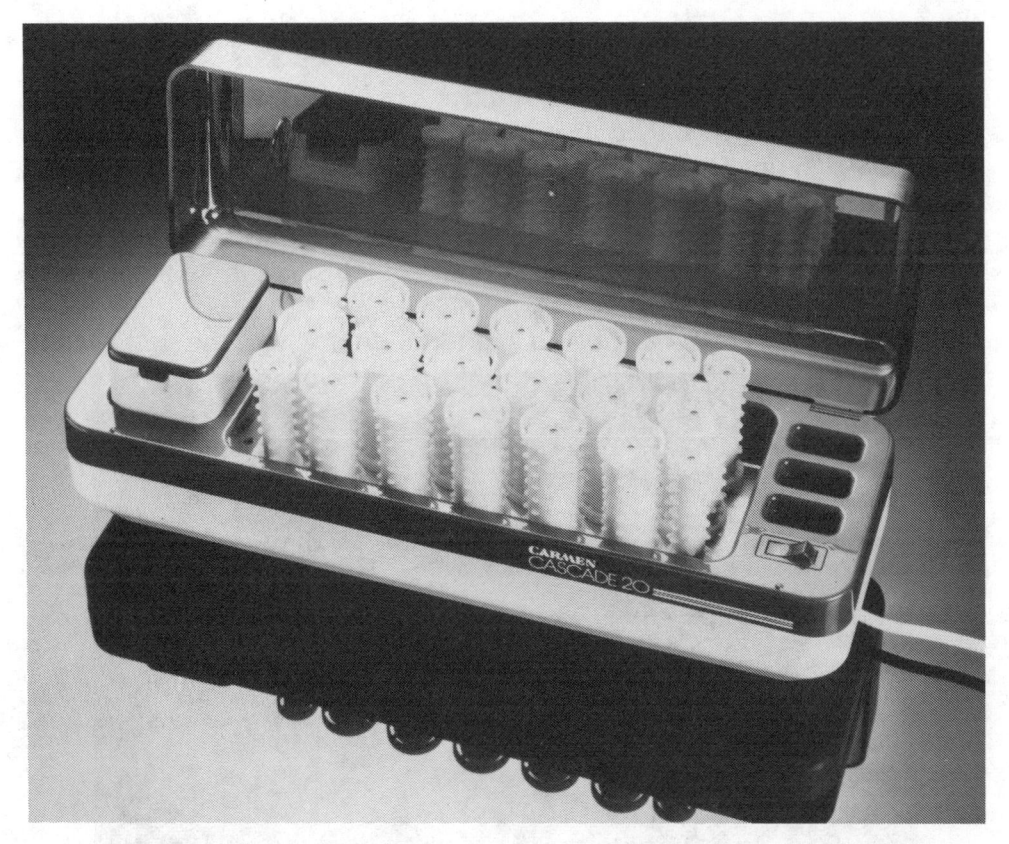

Fig. 3.15 A set of modern heated rollers. (Courtesy of House of Carmen Ltd.)

Heated rollers are put into the hair using the same method as for normal wet setting. However, equally good results can be achieved using slightly larger sections than normal (remember that the number of heated rollers that you have is limited).

If you look at the base of a heated roller you will find that it is colour-coded according to its diameter. Each size has its own colour-coded clip for securing the roller in position. The straight side of the clip should always be as near to the scalp as possible without causing discomfort. Using the wrong size of clip means that eventually the clips will become distorted.

When the rollering is complete, the rollers should be left in the hair until the indicator dot returns back to being red. For best results, leave until the rollers are completely cold. Remove the rollers by gently unwinding each roller (if you have wound up carefully and smoothly, the rollers will be easy to remove) and continue with styling.

Hood driers

Hood driers can be wall-mounted, fitted as a bank, or individually fitted on a pedestal with wheels. The need for hood driers has decreased as blow drying has become more popular and many salons now save space by choosing wall-mounted driers.

Hood driers need to be dusted regularly and the upholstery of the seats should also be cleaned. If a build-up of fluff and dust is allowed to occur, it could shorten the life of the drier.

Figure 3.16 shows an example of a modern drier where the stylist is able

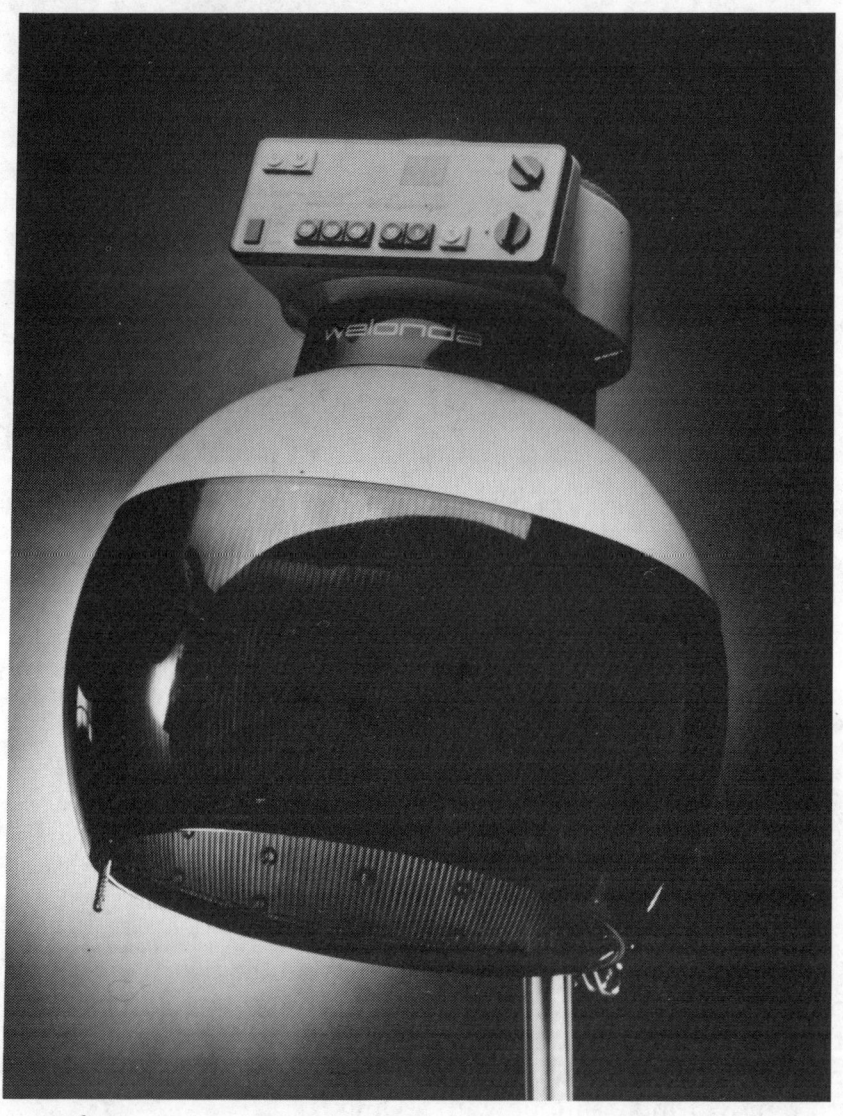

Fig. 3.16 A modern hood drier with its own in-built timer. (Courtesy of Wella Ltd.)

to programme in the required drying time, and set the temperature. A warning 'bleep' indicates when the drying time is about to end.

Climazons and other accelerators

A Climazon is an example of a modern accelerator. They produce infra-red heat which can be used for accelerating chemical processes and for drying styles which would be spoiled if they were disturbed by the moving air of a conventional drier. Climazons are available as pedestal or wall-mounted models.

The manufacturer's instructions should be followed according to the process for which the Climazon is being used. The programming panel tells the operator to key in the appropriate time and gives a warning 'bleep' to indicate when this is about to run out. Other types of accelerator use a number of small infra-red bulbs in a canopy that resembles a hood drier. The octopus uses several large bulbs which could be positioned around the head. Single hand-held models are also available with one large bulb.

Infra-red rays of the wrong frequency can cause cataracts in the eyes, but today's models are usually carefully selected to avoid this. Remember that infra-red radiation is invisible, so it is possible to burn the skin before one is fully aware of the damage being done.

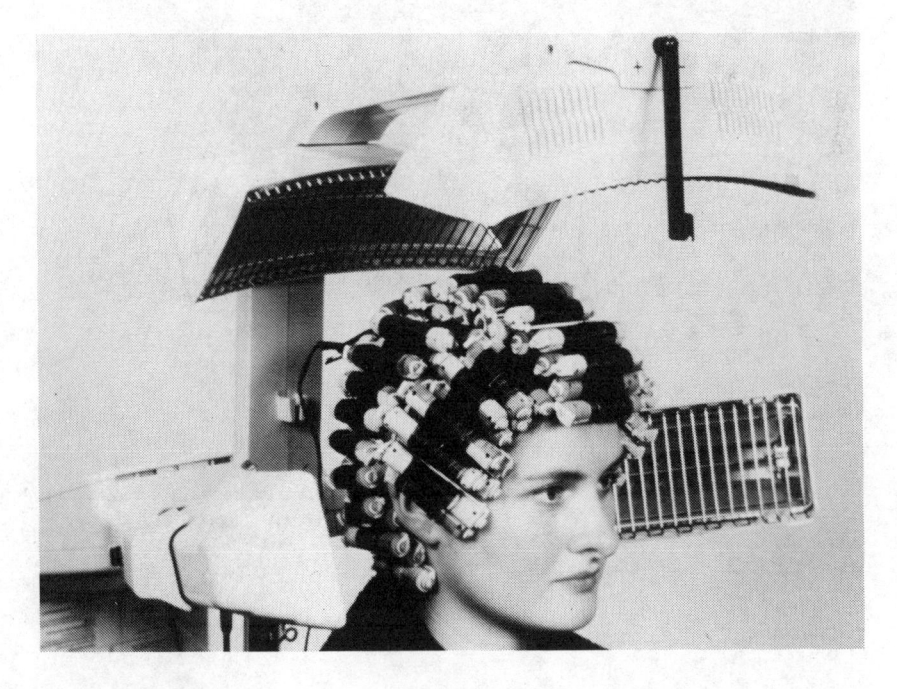

Fig. 3.17 A Climazon. (Courtesy of Wella Ltd.)

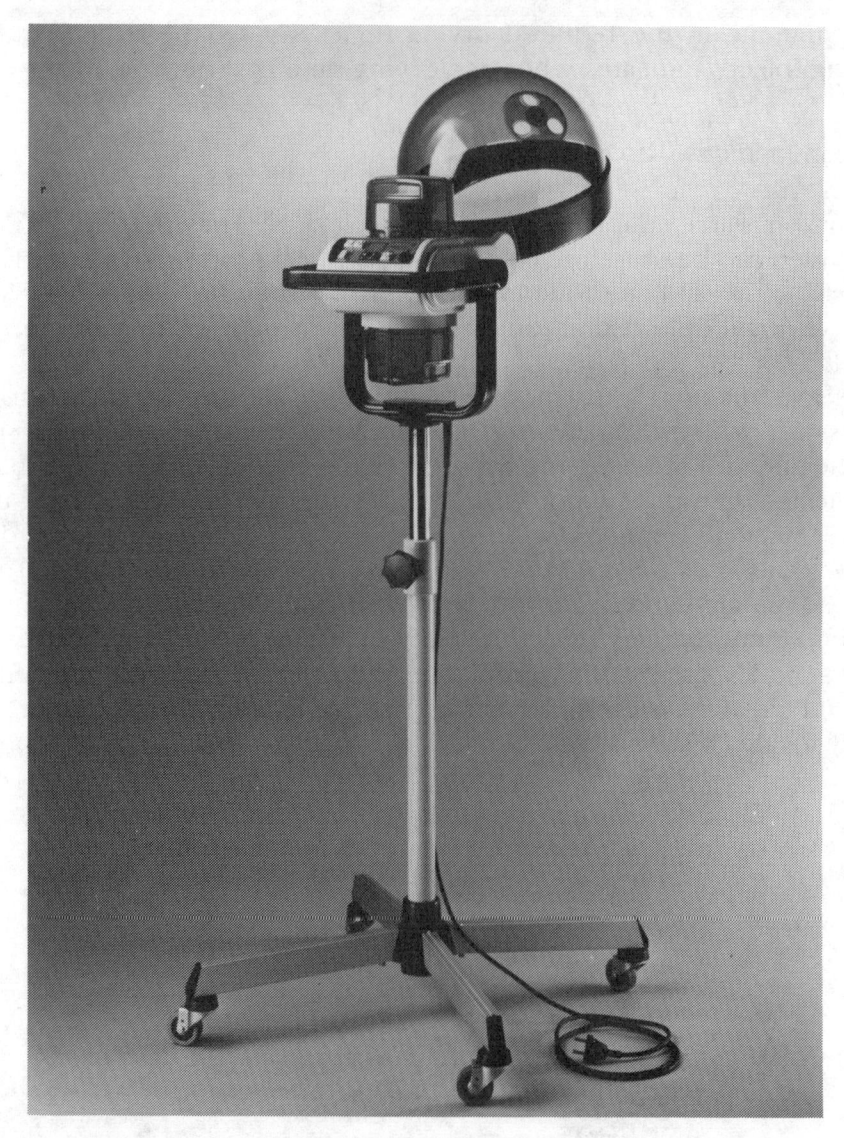

Fig. 3.18 A modern steamer. (Courtesy of Wella Ltd.)

Steamers

Steamers provide moist heat, unlike the dry, moving air, of a hood drier. They do this by producing steam from tiny nozzles inside a plastic dome. Steamers are used as part of hair treatments mainly because the moist heat helps the conditioning product to penetrate the hair shaft. Steamers are particularly good at restoring moisture levels when used on black hair.

Only distilled water should be used in a steamer unless you live in a soft water district or have a water softener fitted in your salon. The dissolved calcium bicarbonate in hard water turns into solid scale, calcium carbonate, when heated up to around 60°C. This blocks the steam nozzles and can stop an expensive machine from working properly, although it is possible to descale steamers in the same way as a kettle or coffee-maker. Steamers should be switched on before they are needed, to give the water time to heat up. Also, check that the cold water reservoir has water in it. The particular model shown in Fig. 3.18 has a built-in timer which gives a warning 'bleep' as the machine is about to switch itself off.

3.3 Hairdressing tools

There is a proverb which says 'a bad workman always blames his tools'. In hairdressing, professional tools should be used to enable the operator to achieve the highest standards possible according to his or her ability. A comb or a pair of scissors bought from the local chemist will not withstand the frequent use encountered in a salon. This is why the major manufacturers produce tools to such high standards. Leave other tools for the 'cowboys' of the trade and equip yourself as well as you can afford. Remember to look after your tools and they will give you years of service.

Clips

A number of different clips are used to hold the hair in place. They are best sterilised in disinfectants. The following are examples of pins and grips:

Hair clamps
This type of clip is used to hold large quantities of hair when the hair needs to be sectioned for particular processes such as perming, cutting or colouring. They are made of plastic and come in a variety of different colours. The top of the clip is squeezed together to open the 'jaws' which

end in short teeth. The jaws will close when the pressure is released from the top of the clip. Figure 3.19 illustrates a hair clamp.

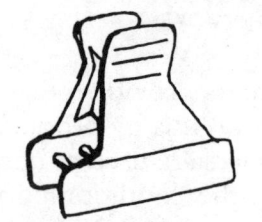

Fig. 3.19 A plastic hair clamp.

Sectioning clips
These are usually made of metal and may be obtained with bright coloured coatings. The long prongs of the clip will hold quite large quantities of hair cleanly out of the way for the stylist. The end of the clip is squeezed together to open the prongs and close once the pressure is released. A sectioning clip is illustrated in Fig. 3.20.

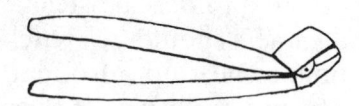

Fig. 3.20 A sectioning clip.

Double-prong clip
These are usually made of metal but plastic ones are also available. This type of clip is smaller than the others previously mentioned and they are not intended to hold large quantities of hair. They are used mainly to secure pincurls (see Chapter 6). Figure 3.21 illustrates a double-prong clip.

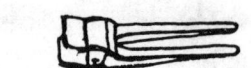

Fig. 3.21 A double-prong clip.

Hairpins and grips

As with hair clips, a number of different types is available for securing rollers or hair in place. They are best sterilised using disinfectants. The following are examples of pins and grips:

Fine wavy pins
These pins are made of metal and are available in several shades to match different hair colours. They can be used to hold hair in place in the final dressing because they are fine, and if the right colour is used, can be effectively concealed in the hair. Fine wavy pins can also be used to secure flat pincurls in position and are preferred by many stylists for this because they do not mark the hair as much as metal double-prong clips. Because they are fine, the prongs are very pliable, with a tendency to bend, so are not effective for holding large quantities of hair securely. A fine wavy pin is illustrated in Fig. 3.22.

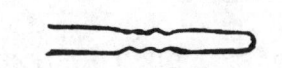

Fig. 3.22 A fine wavy pin.

Straight prong pins

Straight prong pins, otherwise known as setting pins, come in various colours to match the hair. They are also available in different lengths, the most common being 6–7 cms (3 inches) long. Apart from being used to hold rollers in place, they can also be effective for holding hair securely in place when dressing the hair. In the latter case, they would normally be used in conjunction with fine wavy pins. A straight prong pin is illustrated in Fig. 3.23.

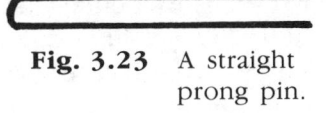

Fig. 3.23 A straight prong pin.

Plastic setting pins

These are often preferred by stylists to the metal pins just described for securing rollers in place. They do, however, have a tendency to distort if they are misused by forcing them into rollers. A plastic setting pin is illustrated in Fig. 3.24.

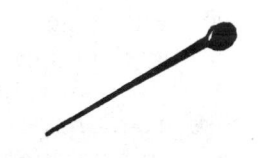

Fig. 3.24 A plastic setting pin.

Hairgrips

These are made of metal and come in a variety of colours. In North America they are called Bobbi pins. They are available in both a shiny and matt finish, the latter being preferred for film and TV work, because they do not glint in bright light. The flat prong is always placed against the scalp as the wavy prong could cause discomfort. The two ends of the prongs are guarded by a plastic covering which resembles a small blob, protecting the client from the otherwise sharp ends. The blobs also make the opening of the grip easier. A hairgrip is illustrated in Fig. 3.25.

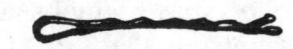

Fig. 3.25 A hairgrip.

Rollers

Rollers are made of either plastic or metal, or a combination of both. They can be either cylindrical or cone-shaped and come in various lengths and diameters. Two are illustrated in Fig. 3.26.

The best type of rollers to use are smooth, because they do not mark the hair when it is wrapped around it. Spiked rollers may be easier to put in (because the hair will grip onto it), but they will mark the hair, especially if it is fine or fragile. Some stylists use a layer of tissue around spiked rollers when setting bleached hair to prevent marking or damage to the hair meshes. Another advantage of using smooth rollers is that they will never tangle in the hair.

There are rollers available which have a circular brush in their centre. They are made of metal wire loops and have a fine mesh covering, through which the bristles protrude. Again, although this helps to grip the hair there is evidence that damage is caused. In the United States it has been shown that these types of rollers can puncture the hair and damage it as it dries.

All rollers have perforations which allow the hair mesh to dry more quickly. Either metal or plastic pins can be used to secure the rollers in place (clips are more popular in the United States) but care should always be taken that the hair wrapped around the roller is not disturbed when it is secured. Rollers are best sterilised in disinfectant or a formaldehyde cabinet. They should be washed frequently.

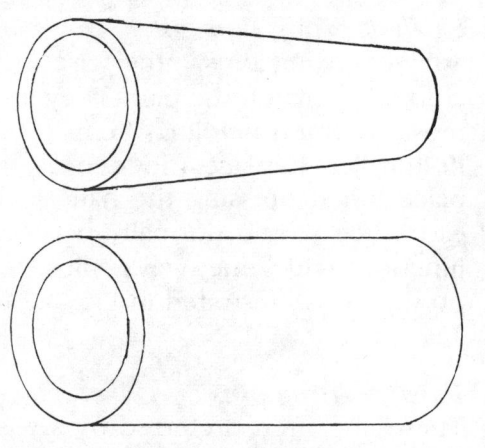

Fig. 3.26 A cylindrical and cone-shaped roller.

Spiral curlers

Spiral curlers are made of plastic and can be used for either setting or perming hair. They come in various lengths and diameters. One is illustrated in Fig. 3.27. The hair is wrapped around the curler and sits in the spiral groove that runs down the entire length of the curler. Special plastic clips are used to fasten the points onto the curler. The result, whether set or permed, will be a ringlet curl.

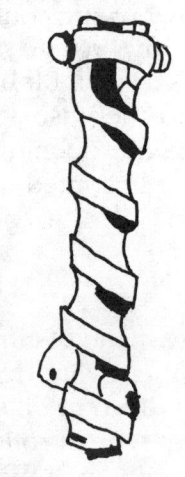

Fig. 3.27 A spiral curler.

Rik-Raks

Rik-Raks are made of plastic which is of a flexible 'V' shape, as shown in Fig. 3.28. A mesh of hair is taken and woven through the two prongs in a figure of eight. The result is a deep wave in a zig-zag pattern. Rik-Raks can be used for setting or perming the hair.

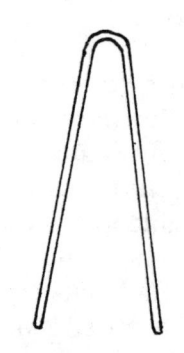

Fig. 3.28 A Rik-Rak.

Molton Browners

The term 'Molton Browners' is now used to refer to many different types of 'rollers' that are available on the market. The original Molton Browners were created by the salon of the same name in London. They were soft, flexible rollers which consisted of a metal wire covered with padding and cloth. The central wire enables the roller to be bent to secure it in position. The hair should be dry for the cloth type of Molton Browner, so they can only be used for setting the hair.

Another type of Molten Browners are made of foam and can be used for both setting or perming hair because they do not absorb moisture from the hair so readily. (Wella market the foam type under the name of Molton Permers.) These also have a central spine of wire which enables them to be bent to stay in place. Figure 3.29 shows both types of Molton Browners, and there are many cheaper copies on the market.

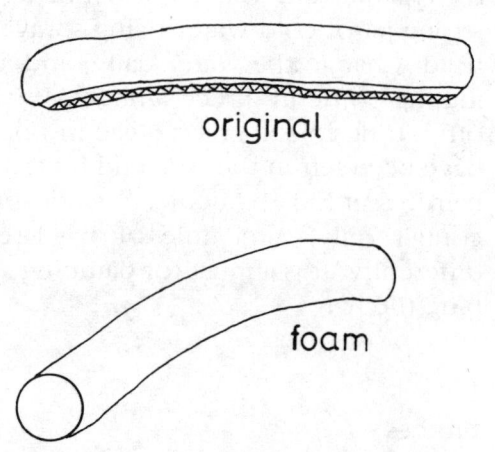

Fig. 3.29 The original cloth-covered Molton Browner (above) and the foam type (underneath).

Mad Mats

Mad Mats resemble flat rectangles of J-cloth which have sponge and wires running through them. They were developed by the Mad Hackers salon in London by Maureen and Kevin Bura. (Mad Mats are also featured in *Perming and Straightening – A Salon Handbook*.) They are reusable and are available in three widths and lengths. They can equally well be used for setting or perming. The hair can be curled, twisted, and even corrugated because Mad Mats can be easily manipulated into any shape. If long hair is being styled, extra Mats can be added. They do not require pins as they can just be bent over to secure the hair in place. A mesh of hair is simply placed on the Mat and it is then folded over.

Water sprays

Water sprays are essential implements in every hairdresser's (and gardener's!) tool kit. Everyone knows what they look like but we have still included one just in case, see Fig. 3.30. The bottle is filled with water and when the trigger is squeezed a sprayed jet or mist of water comes out of the nozzle. By adjusting the nozzle it is possible to adjust the fineness of the spray. Check the spray against your hand to check that it is correctly adjusted. Clients will not appreciate a strong jet of cold water being sprayed on their head! Change the water daily, and avoid leaving the bottle in direct sunlight. It can be very off-putting to see green algae in bottles which have been left in the sun, and it hardly makes a hairdresser look hygienic. A water spray should contain only water unless it has been labelled differently. It is a must for damping and redamping the hair.

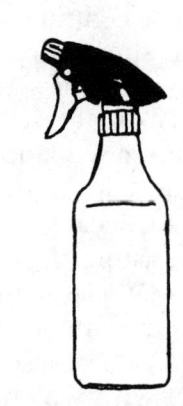

Fig. 3.30 A water spray bottle.

Brushes

An extensive range of brushes is available for the hairdresser to choose from. Some of the brushes mentioned are for specific tasks or styling techniques, while others are more versatile and are used more frequently.

Basically, all brushes are made of bristles, which can be natural hog bristle, nylon or wire. These bristles are embedded into a wooden, plastic or rubber moulded handle. Natural bristles, although more expensive, are best for a brush, because they are made of natural keratin and there is less friction and wear on the hair in use. Natural bristle will also enable the hair to be penetrated, gripped and placed more easily. Nylon bristles are often criticised because of their hardness, as this will wear down the hair more, but the ends of the bristles can be rounded to avoid scratching the scalp and nylon can easily be cleaned and sterilised. Remember, as well, that the client will not be visiting the salon so often that your brush will cause excessive damage. The bristles of a brush must be set into tufts or rows, as this allows the loose or shed hair to collect in the grooves without interfering with the action of the bristles.

What effect has brushing on the hair?

Brushing transfers sebum from the skin along the cuticle of the hair shaft. This coating of oil helps to keep the moisture content of the hair constant at about 10 per cent. The oil reduces the tendency of the hairs to mesh together and tangle or form knots and the right amount of sebum will impart a natural lustre to the hair. It will also stimulate the circulation of the blood and lymph supplies to the scalp, removing waste products more efficiently and promoting hair growth. Brushing also helps remove dead skin cells and debris from the hair, which in turn will discourage the growth of micro-organisms such as bacteria and fungi.

If the sebaceous glands of a client are over-active, brushing will not tend to make the sebaceous glands noticeably more over-active. Brushing should still be carried out, but the hair should be shampooed more regularly. Brushing the hair will help to relax the client as well. The only really detrimental effect is that the hair will tend to become slightly damaged towards the front of the hairline, the cuticle becoming more roughened and the hair therefore becoming more porous.

How do I sterilise hairbrushes?

Before using a brush on a client it should be cleaned of all loose debris such as hairs and thoroughly washed. It should then be sterilised by placing it in a container of disinfectant for ten minutes, or as directed by the manufacturer. Remember that brushes can scratch the skin or take the top off spots, so they do need to be thoroughly sterilised. A formaldehyde cabinet can be used as an alternative, and brushes can be stored before use in an ultra-violet cabinet.

Brushes in common salon use today

Flat brush

This type of brush is probably the most commonly used in salons today. It is illustrated in Fig. 3.31. It can be used for brushing the hair into shape after setting and also for blow drying. A flat brush consists of nylon filaments embedded in a rubber base. The rubber base slides into position on the plastic moulded handle. The rubber base can be removed for cleaning and replacement tufts are available to replace ones which have become worn or damaged.

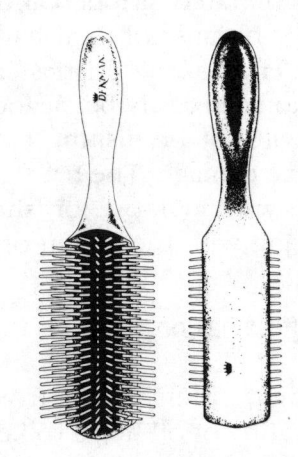

Fig. 3.31 A flat brush, back and front. (Courtesy of Denman.)

Vent brush

These are relative newcomers to the professional market, becoming available for the first time in the 1970s. They have open spaces along the back which allows the airflow from a drier to pass through – hence the alternative name of 'airflow brush'. The nylon tuft filaments are arranged in pairs, a shorter and longer one being embedded into the brush together. As the brush is drawn through the hair, the short and long filaments give the hair a broken, casual texture. If the particular hair being blow dried has a slight natural movement, this will be increased when using a vent brush, because the airflow through the brush increases the hair's natural tendency to curl.

Vent brushes are also very useful during a haircut, as the hair will fall into position allowing the stylist to identify any corrections to the cut that need to be made. A vent brush is shown in Fig. 3.32.

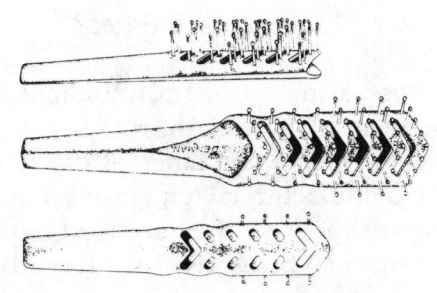

Fig. 3.32 A vent brush, from three viewpoints. (Courtesy of Denman.)

Equipment and Tools

Circular brushes
These come in a variety of different diameters varying from 1–6 cms. The tufts can be either bristle, nylon or a mixture of both. Circular brushes tend to be used only when blow drying. The diameter of the brush will determine how much volume and movement are put into the hair. A small diameter brush will put more curl into the hair than a larger one, in exactly the same way as this principle applies to roller sizes.

Perhaps the most popular range of circular brushes are those designed by Harold Leighton, known as Harold Leighton Stylers. They are exceptionally durable and can be taken apart for cleaning. Several brushes make up the range, and they are ideal to retail in the salon. A circular brush is shown in Fig. 3.33.

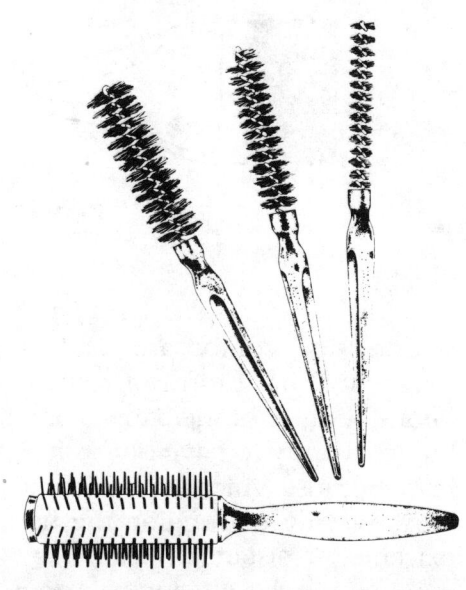

Fig. 3.33 Types of circular brush. (Courtesy of Denman.)

Neck brush
The neck brush is used to clean hair clippings away from the face and neck. It is important that the bristles are long and soft, so that they do not cause discomfort to the client. Putting a little talcum powder on the brush will make wet hair clippings easier to remove from the skin. Use a neck brush repeatedly during a haircut to ensure client comfort. One is illustrated in Fig. 3.34.

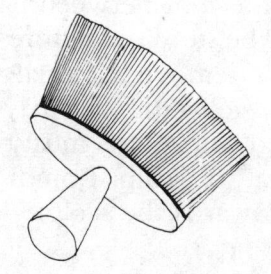

Fig. 3.34 A neck brush.

Tint brush
This is a flat brush with a long narrow handle. The pointed end of the brush can be used to part the hair into sections when colouring the hair. The most expensive tint brushes have softer and closer tufts than the cheaper ones, helping to hold the product on the brush and being kinder

to the client's scalp (they are less likely to scratch the scalp). Tint brushes can also be used to apply conditioner. One is illustrated in Fig. 3.35.

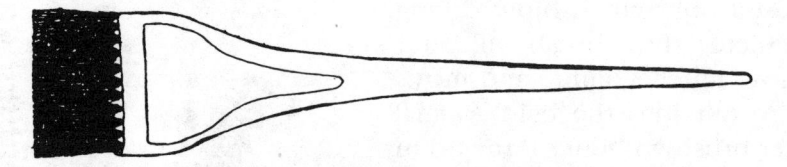

Fig. 3.35 A tint brush.

Combs

Hairdressing combs are made from either nylon, plastic, vulcanite (a toughened, hard form of rubber) or metal. Metal combs are restricted in salons because of the damaging effects they can have on the hair and scalp but it is handy to have one as it can help remove static electricity from the hair. Because vulcanite combs are resistant to heat they are ideal when blow waving or tonging the hair. Some newer types of plastic are also extremely resistant to heat.

When purchasing combs, run your finger along the edge of the teeth, to see if they would scratch the scalp. The teeth of a good comb should have rounded points, with a fine taper and space between them where they join at the base. Avoid combs that pinch the hair at the base of the teeth, as these will tend to pull and tug the hair. Discard any combs which have damaged or missing teeth.

Combs should be regularly cleaned with hot soapy water and sterilised in disinfectant between clients. If you drop combs (or other tools!) they should be sterilised before further use on a client – wiping them on a towel will not remove bacteria!

Damage to the hair may follow the incorrect combing of snarled up or knotted hair. Knots must be separated without undue effort or tugging on the shaft or scalp. Combing should commence at the ends and progress back towards the scalp.

Uses of combing

Combing will remove dead skin scales and debris from the scalp and hair. It also separates the hair into parallel strands which can be gathered into meshes of the required size. Combing can also remove excess water from the hair after it has been shampooed or rinsed. Tints and various creams can be distributed along the hair shaft by the comb, so that the application is evenly applied. A comb is invaluable for parting hair in a preliminary examination of the scalp to check for possible scalp conditions.

Combs in common salon use today

Tail combs

There are two types of tail combs from which a stylist can choose. One has a plastic 'tail' while the other has one made of metal. The metal-ended comb has a much finer end and is particularly useful when dividing the hair into fine sections, such as for perming or weave colouring. It is usually referred to as a 'needle' or 'pin-tail' comb, although in the United States they refer to it as a 'rat-tail' comb. Tail combs usually have only one size of teeth and are used primarily for sectioning the hair, as in setting, perming and weaving. The two types are illustrated in Fig. 3.36.

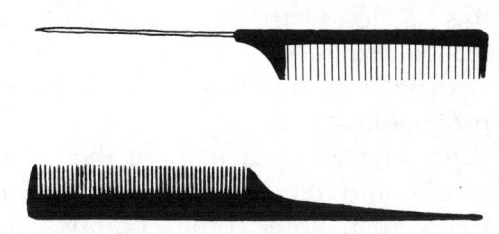

Fig. 3.36 The two main types of tail comb.

Straight combs

These usually have two sizes of teeth and have no tail for making sections. Straight combs come in various sizes, the larger ones being used for disentangling and combing through tints. The more widely spaced teeth prevent pulling on the hair.

They are also used when cutting or dressing the hair after setting. Using a tail comb for this purpose has the disadvantage of having only one size of teeth. With a straight comb you can alternate between backcombing with the fine teeth and smoothing out with the larger teeth. Smaller teeth would drag out the backcombing when smoothing out the hair during dressing.

For certain cutting techniques, extra flexible straight combs are needed. An example is scissor over comb cutting, when a flexible thin comb is needed because it will bend according to the contours of the head, allowing the stylist to achieve a close cut. A straight comb is illustrated in Fig. 3.37.

Fig. 3.37 A straight comb.

All-purpose

All-purpose combs have widely spaced teeth and a large handle. Because of the wide tooth spacing they are not used for styling, but are used for disentangling and combing products (such as tint and conditioners) through the hair. An all-purpose comb is illustrated in Fig. 3.38.

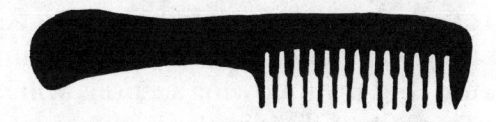

Fig. 3.38 An all-purpose comb.

Afro comb

This has long prong-like teeth made of metal or plastic set into a handle. The teeth are widely spaced because Afro hair is super-curly and ordinary combs would damage the hair. Many people with permed hair who dry it naturally find this type of comb invaluable. In use, the comb is inserted into the hair and used in a 'picking' action and this has led to the term 'hair pick'. Metal blades are more damaging to the hair; alternative materials are therefore preferable.

Because of the length of the teeth the Afro comb tends to be damaged more easily than some other combs. One is illustrated in Fig. 3.39.

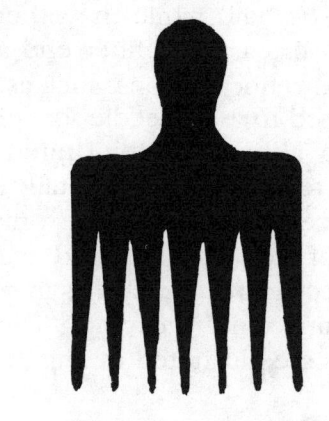

Fig. 3.39 An Afro comb.

3.4 Haircutting tools

These can be divided into different types of scissors, clippers and razors. (We have already discussed electric clippers in [3.2].) They are also the most likely to draw blood, and as such, are the most important implements to sterilise. Every time your tools draw blood they should be sterilised, and this can be achieved with a variety of disinfectants within about 10 minutes without harming your precious tools. Be wary of placing your cutting tools into a formaldehyde cabinet as the vapours can attack and spoil metal. Instead, use ultra-violet cabinets as a handy storage area for your disinfected scissors. If you wish to work professionally, to the highest standards of hygiene, it is necessary to have two sets of cutting tools. Thus you always will have a spare while the other is being disinfected or has been sent off for sharpening. *The recommended method of sterilisation is with an autoclave (type of pressure cooker).*

Scissors

Scissors can be the most expensive non-electrical tools in the salon. Prices range from a few pounds to hundreds. As you will be using them for much of your working life you must have a pair that you use effortlessly, as if they were an extension of your hands. They vary in design and intended use, and the following sections will take us through different scissor types. To work at their peak all scissors should be sharp; just how sharp can be seen from Fig. 3.40.

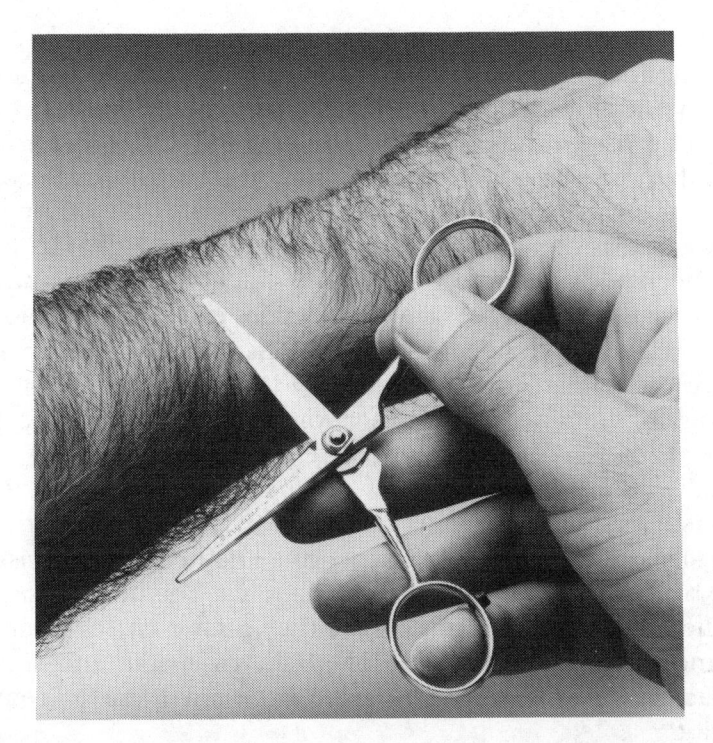

Fig. 3.40 A pair of scissors should be sharp. This pair of Jaguar Perfects can take the hair off an arm. (Courtesy of Rand Rocket Ltd.)

If cutting tools are not sharp, they can damage the hair. This can clearly be seen from Fig. 3.41 (a), (b) and (c). Good quality scissors will be made of well-tempered stainless or cobalt steel and have free-moving, sharp-edged

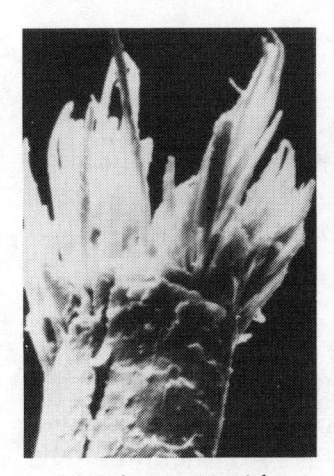

(a) A hair cut with blunt scissors.

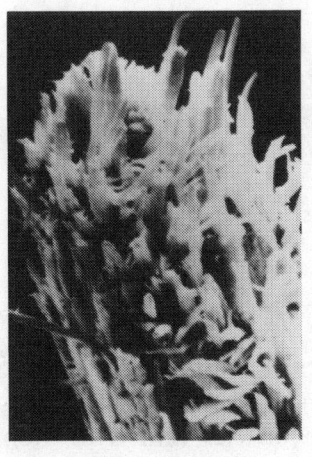

(b) A hair cut with a blunt razor.

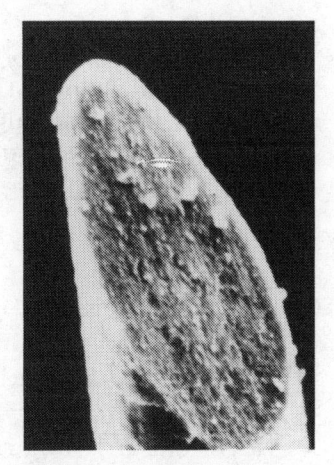

(c) A hair cut with a sharp razor.

Fig. 3.41 (Courtesy of Wella).

blades. Scissors are available in different sizes ranging between 10 cms and 18 cms in length from the tip of the blades to the handles. The size a stylist chooses to work with depends on whichever type feels most comfortable and easy to control for the particular job being done. It is therefore usual to have more than one size in your kit so that you can alternate as the work you are doing changes.

The various parts of a pair of scissors are shown in Fig. 3.42. Usually the points of the blades become blunt most quickly, because these are the parts which are used the most. The blade edges can either be micro-serated or plain, some scissors having one type of each blade. The serrated edges tend to stop the hair from slipping during the closing of the blades when hair is being cut. The pivot of the scissors is usually a fixed screw which cannot be loosened or tightened, except when being sharpened professionally. Some manufacturers are now replacing this screw with more sophisticated arrangements which allow for adjustment to prevent premature slackening of the blades' action. The heel of the scissors is the part of the blades which are nearest the handles. The heel is used for taper cutting. The shanks can be made of either plastic or metal and vary in length. Handles can also be made of plastic or metal, and some have a cushion pad made of rubber or plastic between them to reduce noise when cutting.

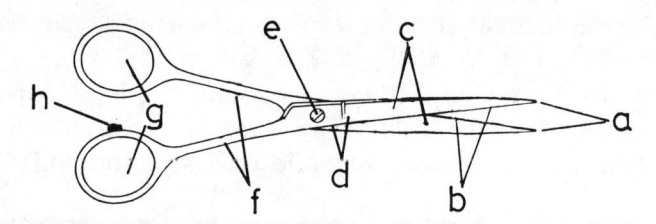

Fig. 3.42 The parts of a pair of scissors.
(a) Points of blades.
(b) Blade edges (can be plain or micro-serrated).
(c) Blades. (d) Heel. (e) Pivot. (f) Shanks. (g) Handles. (h) Cushion pad.

Caring for your scissors

- Wipe the scissor blades clean with a piece of cotton wool or tissue after each use to remove moisture and hair clippings, then sterilise them.
- Never cut anything other than hair with them or they will blunt more quickly.
- Never drop your scissors. It can upset their balance and performance. Carry them in their original protective case.

- Do not lend your scissors to others.
- If the blades do not move easily, try placing some high quality oil between the blades at the base of the handles.
- Always have them sharpened professionally – trade journals will carry advertisements for this.

How are scissors held?

All hairdressing scissors are held with the thumb and third finger as shown in Fig. 3.43(a). This method of handling enables the operator to have maximum control over the scissors. When the scissors are not actually cutting, the thumb should be slipped out of the handle so that the scissors are cradled in the hand while still being supported by the third finger through the handle. By releasing the thumb from the handle the stylist has the manoeuvrability to hold a comb in the same hand, while ensuring that the scissor blades are not open. This is shown in Fig. 3.43(b).

Only the thumb moves when using scissors. Do not have the handle too far down on the thumb or it will restrict your freedom of movement. Spend time handling scissors before you attempt a haircut. Open and close them using only your thumb, one blade remaining stationary while the other moves against it. Also, practise releasing and putting your thumb through the handle, holding a comb in the same hand as your scissors.

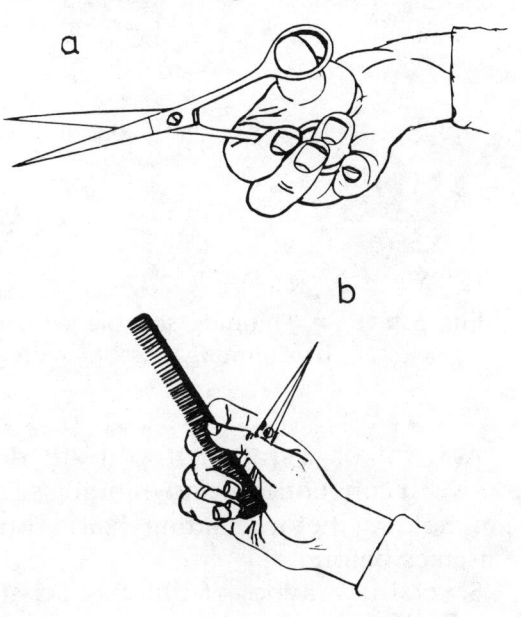

Fig. 3.43 (a) How to hold a pair of scissors correctly. (b) Holding a scissors and comb at the same time.

Thinning scissors

There are two main types of thinning scissors; those which have both blades notched, and those which have one ordinary blade and one notched blade. Thinning scissors may also sometimes be described in the following terms:

- aescalup
- texturising scissors
- serrated scissors
- notched scissors.

Perhaps it is because thinning scissors have become popular again recently that the trade feels they should be referred to by more up-to-date names! Thinning scissors with two notched blades will remove less hair than a pair with one plain and one notched blade (see Fig. 5.10). The two types of thinning scissors are shown in Fig. 3.44.

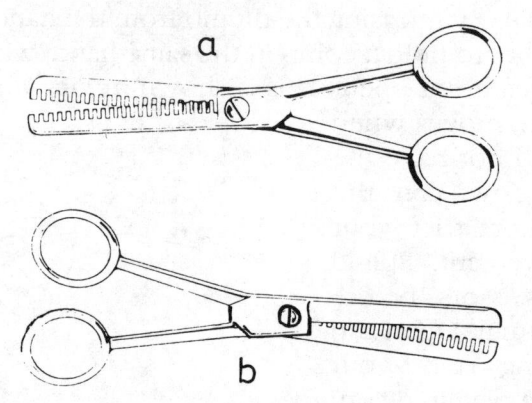

Fig. 3.44 (a) Thinning scissors with two notched blades.
(b) Thinning scissors with one plain and one notched blade.

A word of warning! If you are doing a haircut and are alternating between conventional and thinning scissors, always check which ones you are holding before cutting hair with them. We have witnessed such mistakes before!

Several new types of thinning scissors have been developed recently. The notched blades are now available with wider and narrower spaces between the teeth. These types of scissors are used to create various degrees of texture throughout a haircut. Some people argue that a good haircutter requires only one pair of conventional scissors to achieve the same results, but the advantage of the special scissors is that all-important commodity – time. It takes a long time pointing out or weave cutting hair, and this type of scissors makes the job a lot quicker. Figure 3.45 shows two pairs of such special thinning scissors.

Scissors with interchangeable blades are also available. Three different types are shown in Fig. 3.46, while Fig. 3.47 shows the result when used

Equipment and Tools 73

on the hair. These can achieve accurate cutting results in one snip of the scissors.

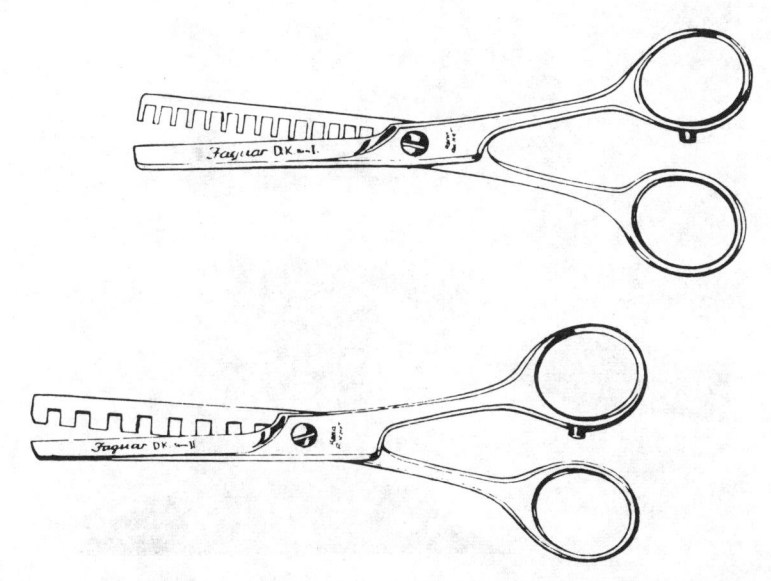

Fig. 3.45 Thinning scissors with different spaces between the teeth can be used to texture the hair quickly. (Courtesy of Rand Rocket Ltd.)

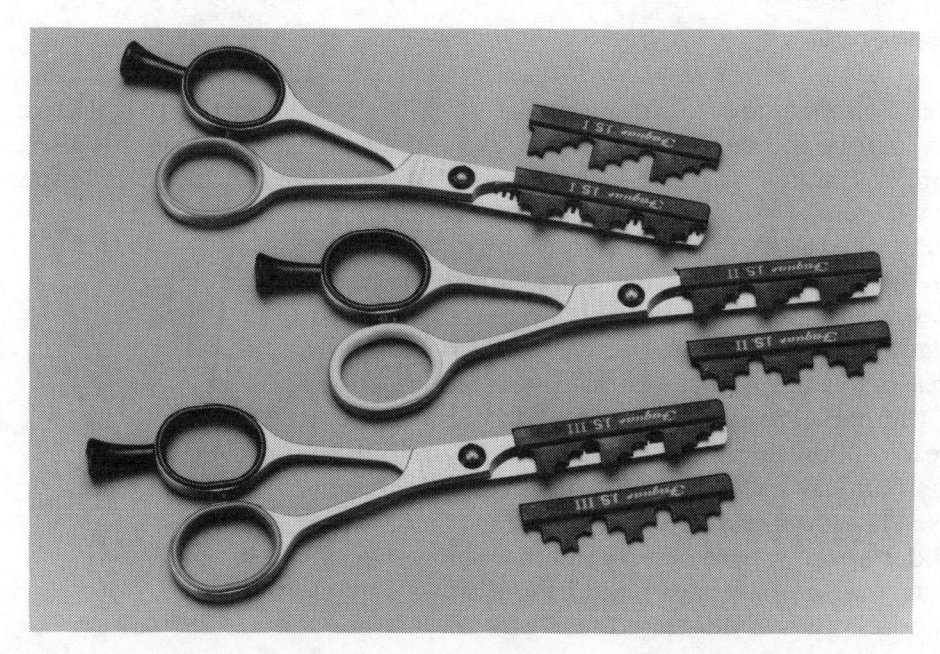

Fig. 3.46 Scissors with interchangeable blades can be used to create a variety of different effects when cutting hair. These are the Jaguar Detour Stylers, showing J.S.I., II and III attachments. The scissors have a removable finger rest. (Courtesy of Rand Rocket Ltd.)

74 Cutting and Styling: a salon handbook

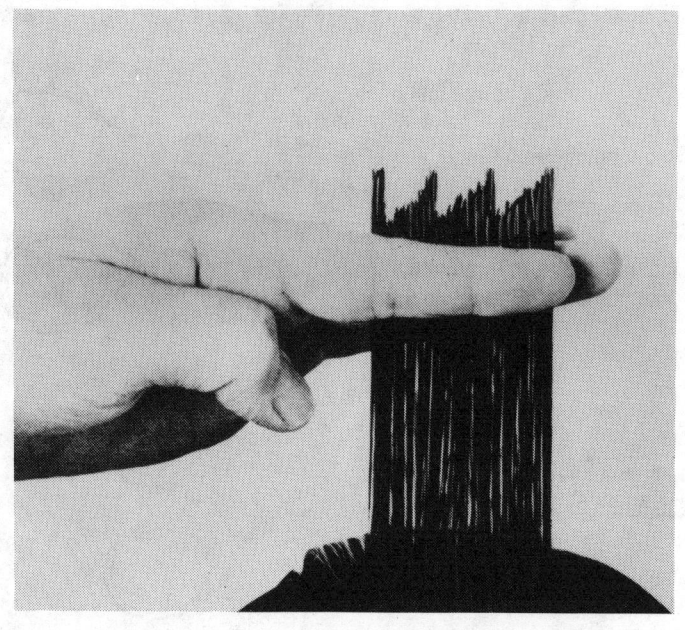

Fig. 3.47 Point cutting of hair achieved in a single snip by using the Jaguar Detour Stylers J.S.II. (Courtesy of Rand Rocket Ltd.)

Hand clippers

Hand clippers are not frequently used in the salon because of the greater popularity and extra safety of electric clippers. Their portability is also no longer unique with the development of rechargeable electric clippers. Hand clippers are operated by squeezing the handles together, making the movable upper blade move across the fixed blade underneath. It is the distance between the points of the two blades and the spacing between the blade teeth that determine the closeness of the hair cut.

Clippers are available with different cutting heads, 0000 being the finest. If clippers pull on the hair, try cleaning and adjusting them. Never use clippers if any of the teeth are broken as the wider spacing between the teeth could result in dragging the hair and cutting the skin. A pair of hand clippers is illustrated in Fig. 3.48.

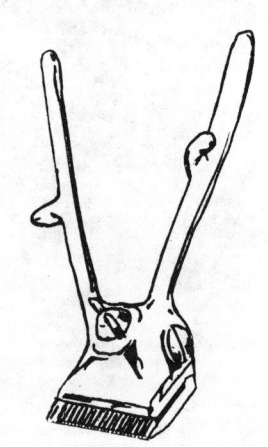

Fig. 3.48 A pair of hand clippers.

Razors

The razors used in hairdressing either have a fixed blade that must be sharpened or a replaceable blade. Open, or cut-throat razors can be either hollow-ground or solid-ground. A cut-throat razor is illustrated in Fig. 3.49(a).

The hollow-ground or German type is generally preferred by hairdressers for shaving. As the name implies, a hollow-ground razor has a hollow appearance between the edge and the back of the razor (see Fig. 3.49(b)) and is made of a softer steel. A solid-ground or French razor has a different wedge-shaped blade and is the preferred razor for razor-cutting hair. The blade shape is shown in Fig. 3.49(c).

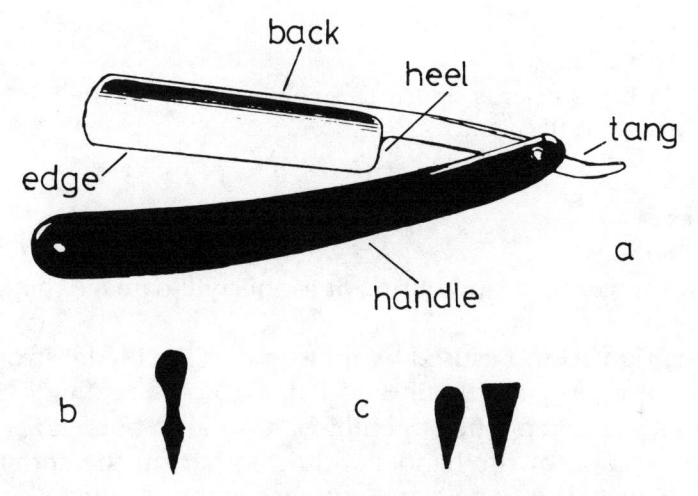

Fig. 3.49 (a) The parts of a cut-throat razor.
(b) Cross section of a hollow-ground blade.
(c) Cross section of a solid-ground blade.

Hair shapers

Hair shapers are very similar to the cut-throat razor except that they have separate disposable blades. A hair shaper also has a metal guard which covers the cutting edge of the blade. Some hair shapers have a straight handle which is not used as a cover for the blade edge. The castellated guard-bar can be left on or taken off for shaping the hair. The hair shaper can also be used for shaving. The hair shaper illustrated in Fig. 3.50 has its guard in place.

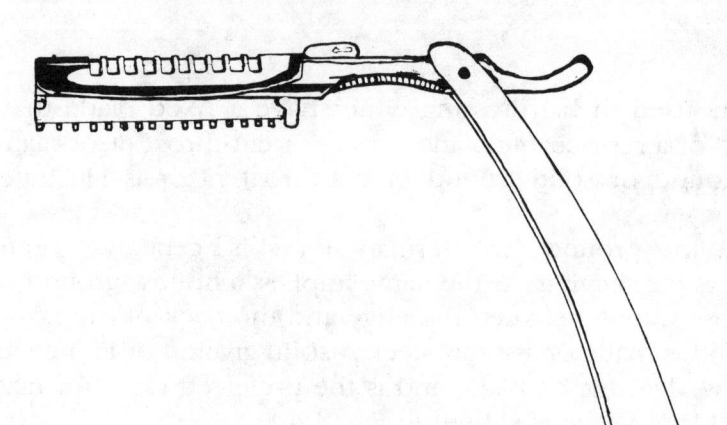

Fig. 3.50 A hair shaper is similar to a conventional open razor but uses a disposable blade.

Care of razors

- Be careful never to drop your razor as this will damage the fine cutting edge.
- To prevent corrosion caused by moisture on the blade, strop the razor after use and apply a little fine oil.
- Care should be taken when opening or closing an open razor. Keep one hand at the base of the handle and the other on the shoulder of the razor. This way the fingers are kept away from the razor edge.

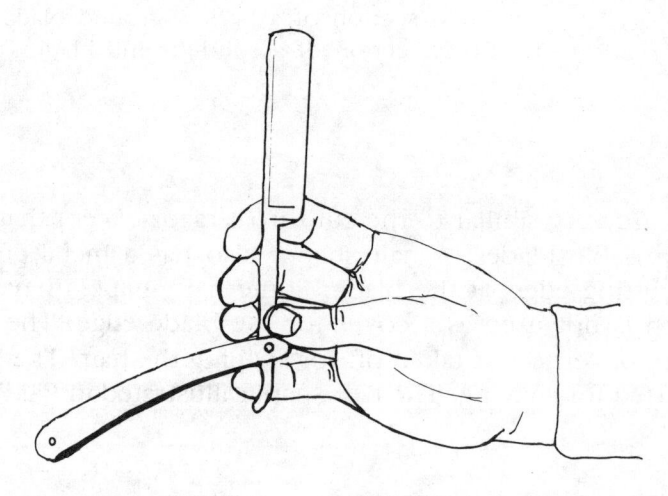

Fig. 3.51 How a razor should be held.

- Hold the open razor with the thumb on the underside of the shank and the little finger resting on top of the tang. The other fingers should rest on top of the shank, as shown in Fig. 3.51. You should be able to hold the razor firmly with this particular grip, so that it can move freely in all directions.
- Razors will require setting to maintain them. This involves the processes of honing and stropping. Honing is carried out to remove damage to the blade edge or to sharpen blades which have become exceptionally blunt. The stropping then maintains the sharpness of the blade.

Honing razors

Two types of hone are available – natural or synthetic. Natural hones include slate, water and Belgian oilstones; these have a fine texture and a smooth surface. Synthetic hones include the carborundum stone and Indian hone; these have a coarse texture and a rougher surface. You can check for damage to the edge of a blade by running it gently against the edge of your thumb nail, a damaged blade will run unevenly against your nail.

If a blade is damaged it will require honing on a synthetic stone first to remove the damage quickly, followed by honing on a natural hone to get a fine edge to the blade (this is rather like rubbing down paintwork with coarse sandpaper to remove the paint, followed by fine sandpaper to prepare the surface for painting). Before honing commences, the surface of the hone should be lubricated with some water, spirit or oil, depending on its type. Then place the hone on a solid surface of a suitable height. The method of honing varies according to whether you are setting a hollow- or solid-ground blade.

Hollow-ground
Place the blade flat against the hone. Exerting equal pressure with each stroke, move the blade over the hone surface in a figure of eight. To turn the razor over at the end of this movement, so that the other side of the blade can be honed, turn the *razor* over and *not* your wrist. This will help ensure that equal pressure is exerted. Give both sides of the blade an equal number of strokes, decreasing the pressure with the last few strokes (see Fig. 3.52 for how to hone a hollow-ground razor). Finish off the honing with a couple of single strokes each way.

Test the blade for sharpness by *gently* drawing the side of the blade edge across the moistened ball of your thumb, it should 'bite' or 'grip' the skin if it has a keen edge. This is due to the tiny 'saw teeth' that you have imparted to the blade edge during honing. They will eventually help grip

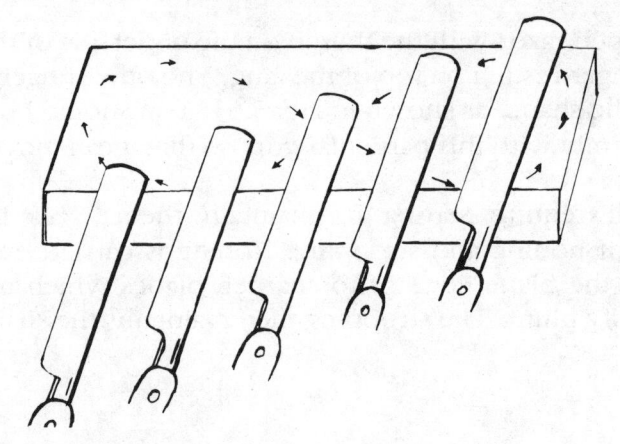

Fig. 3.52 Honing a hollow-ground razor. Turn the blade at the end of each stroke and not the wrist. If the same pressure is exerted on each stroke the sides of the blade will be set at the same angle. If the pressure differs, one side of the blade edge will be worn more than the other.

the hair while cutting or shaving. A blade which is not sharp will run smoothly against the skin.

Solid-ground

Because a solid-ground or French razor is made of a softer steel, less pressure needs to be used when honing. The blade of the razor is placed flat on one end of the hone, with its blade edge pointing towards the centre of the hone. It is then slid, exerting little pressure, *across* and *along* the hone. The blade is then turned over, and the same procedure is carried out from the other end of the hone. You will be producing movements that make a 'V' towards the centre of the hone, as illustrated in Fig. 3.53. Less strokes will be required to produce a keen edge. The strokes should eventually be made starting more towards the centre of the hone so that a smaller V is produced. The blade can be held slightly upright as honing finishes. Check against the moistened ball of the thumb for sharpness.

Fig. 3.53 Honing a solid-ground or French razor. The movements across the hone should make a 'V' shaped movement.

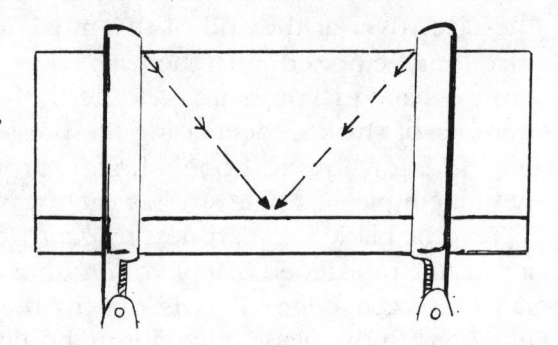

Equipment and Tools   79

The razor is now ready for stropping
Hollow-ground razors require a hanging strop which has one side made of canvas and the other side made of leather. Dry soap is used as a dressing for the canvas side and it is rubbed in using the side of a glass bottle. The leather side is gently scraped with a blunt knife to remove any old dressing and then either oil or tallow is rubbed in with the side of a glass bottle.

The strop used for solid-ground or French razors is called a hand strop. It consists of a piece of wood with a handle; this has leather on one side and balsa wood on the other. The dressing used on the leather and balsa wood is called 'Hamon paste', and this has a gentle abrasive action. There are two grades of Hamon paste, the finer one being used on the leather. The paste is used sparingly to avoid a build-up on the surface of the leather or balsa wood.

Stropping a hollow-ground razor
The strop, secured to the wall at one end, is held outright by one hand so that it is taut. The blade is first cleaned on the canvas side of the strop. The blade is then placed flat against the leather at the top of the strop, with the edge of the razor facing *away* from the centre of the strop. The blade is then gently drawn down the strop, turned over, and pushed up the opposite way. This is illustrated in Fig. 3.54. After several strokes the razor should now be extremely sharp. This can be tested by taking a single hair between the fingers and cutting it with the razor. If it is sharp, the blade will cut the hair without 'pushing' it.

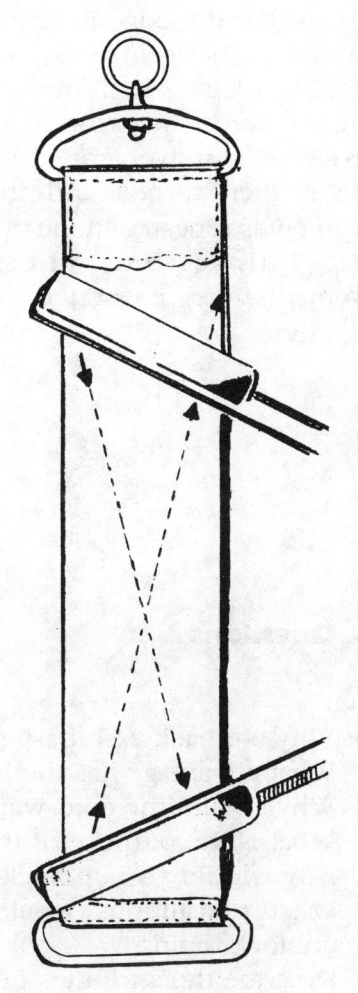

Fig. 3.54 Stropping a hollow-ground razor.

Stropping a solid-ground razor

The strop is placed on a level surface and a few strokes are made on the balsa wood, as described below, to align the teeth that have been formed when honing. The balsa wood is used first because it is covered with the more abrasive Hamon paste. The hand strop is now turned with the leather side up. The blade of the razor is placed against the leather side of the strop so that the edge is facing away from the centre of the strop. The blade is then pushed along and across the strop in an inverted 'V' movement. The blade is then turned and the movement is repeated in the opposite direction. These movements are illustrated in Fig. 3.55.

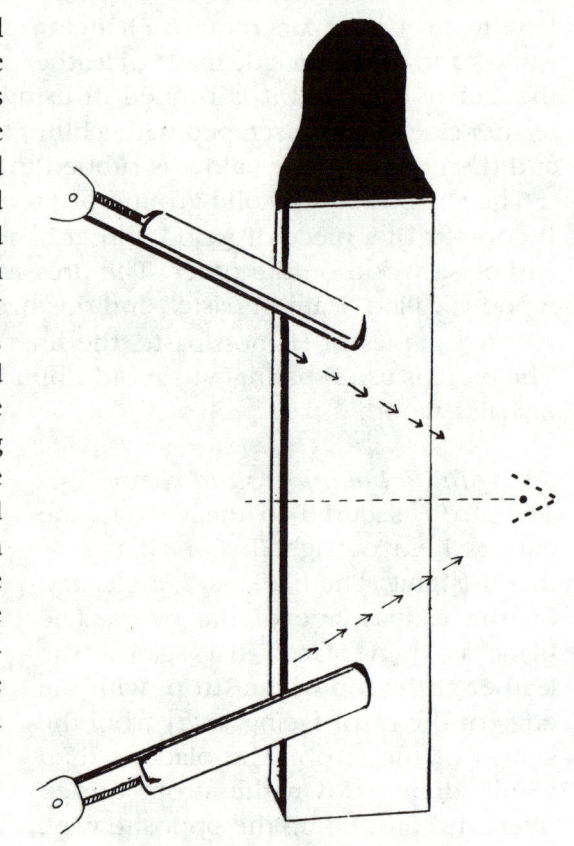

Fig. 3.55 Stropping a solid-ground or French razor on a hand strop.

3.5 Questions

1. Why are backwash basins preferred to forward wash ones?
2. What advantage has the island arrangement for basins?
3. Why should the cold water be turned on first with a mixer tap?
4. What is the purpose of the trap underneath a sink?
5. How would you unblock a trap?
6. What precautions would you take when using caustic soda to unblock drains?
7. Describe the attributes of a modern salon chair.
8. Why should electrical appliances have a British Standards number?
9. What features should a salon hairdrier have?

Equipment and Tools

10 Why do hairdriers have a filter?
11 How can you vary the airflow of a hairdrier?
12 List the safe working guidelines of a hairdrier.
13 Why are hot brushes preferred by many people to tongs?
14 How long do you hold the hot brush in the mesh of hair?
15 What is an 'independent hotbrush'?
16 Why is the safety tip a useful feature in electric curling tongs?
17 How would you protect the scalp from heat when using tongs?
18 List the main points of the safe working guidelines for tongs.
19 How do New Wave tongs differ from normal curling tongs?
20 How and when would you use crimpers?
21 What is the difference between crimpers and the Wave Maker?
22 On what type of hair would you use a straightener?
23 How do electric clippers cut hair?
24 What should you do to the clippers if you cut someone with them?
25 How do you know that your heated rollers are ready?
26 How long should the rollers be left in the hair?
27 When would you use a Climazon or accelerator?
28 When would you use a steamer?
29 What type of water would you use in a steamer?
30 What use has an in-built timer?
31 Describe the use of hair clamps.
32 Describe the use of sectioning clips.
33 When would you use a double-prong clip?
34 How would you secure a roller in place?
35 When would you use a straight prong pin?
36 Describe how you would use a hairgrip.
37 What are the two different shapes of roller?
38 Why are smooth rollers the best ones to use?
39 How can spiked rollers damage hair and how do some stylists prevent this?
40 What are spiral curlers used for?
41 What is a Rik-Rak?
42 How are Molton Browners used?
43 What are Mad Mats and what can you use them for?
44 Why should you regularly change the water in a water spray?
45 Describe the different types of bristles used in hairbrushes.
46 Why is natural bristle preferred to nylon?
47 What is a flat brush and what is it used for?
48 What is a vent brush and what is it used for?
49 When would you use circular brushes?
50 When should you use a neck brush?
51 What is a tint brush and when would you use it?

82 Cutting and Styling: a salon handbook

52 What are combs made from?
53 How can a comb damage the hair?
54 What uses has combing compared to brushing?
55 What is a tail comb and when would you use one?
56 What is a straight comb and what advantage has it over a tail comb?
57 How is an all-purpose comb similar to a tail comb?
58 On what type of hair would you use an Afro comb?
59 How does the combing action of an Afro comb differ from a normal comb?
60 How and when would you sterilise your cutting tools?
61 Why should scissors be sharp?
62 What advantage has a serrated blade?
63 How are scissors held?
64 What are thinning scissors?
65 What advantage do thinning scissors have over conventional scissors for pointing or weave cutting hair?
66 Why should you not use clippers with damaged teeth?
67 What is the difference between a hollow-ground and a solid-ground blade?
68 What is a hair shaper?
69 What is razor setting?
70 How is this carried out on a hollow-ground blade?
71 How is this carried out on a solid-ground blade?
72 When would you use natural and synthetic hones?
73 How would you check a blade for damage?
74 What two ways are there to check blade sharpness?
75 What is the difference between a hanging and a hand strop?

4
Design Analysis and Preparation

This chapter is concerned with how you assess the needs of your clients and prepare them for subsequent treatment after they have entered your salon. Together, with each client, you must use your professional judgement to evaluate and meet each individual's needs, to give them the *right look*. This look is often referred to as the 'total look' because it should take everything about the client into consideration; the face shape, clothes, job and lifestyle.

4.1 The need for consultation between client and stylist

After greeting the client at reception, they should either be asked to wait there or be given a seat at a styling unit, ready to be seen by their stylist. Clients should not be taken straight through to have their hair shampooed before they have fully discussed their needs with the stylist, no matter how familiar the stylist is with the client's hair. Time spent in an initial discussion is just as important as the time that will be spent actually working on the client with the hands. It is in the initial discussion or negotiations that the client and stylist reach agreement about the look that they are *both* aiming to achieve. If this is misinterpreted, it is unlikely that the client will leave the salon feeling comfortable with her look.

Why should the consultation be at the beginning of an appointment?

There are many technical reasons for this, which are as follows:

- Once the hair has been shampooed, wet and combed straight back

from the face, it is very difficult to envisage the client's existing hair style and how well it was managed.
- The texture and condition of the hair is more difficult to assess once it is wet (you will also have lost the opportunity to have suggested an appropriate hair treatment).
- The hair may need other services that you had not anticipated, such as a perm or relaxer to achieve the desired look, so that the hair would have to be prepared in a particular way. Remember the 70 per cent of clients who are lukewarm when offered further services (see Chapter 2)?
- If you were the stylist who last did the client's hair, you will be able to ask how well it had lasted and how easy it had been to manage? The answers to these questions may tell you how to improve your service to the client by highlighting any weaknesses in your work or hairdressing techniques.
- The clients will know and appreciate that you are giving them a professional service. They expect personal attention and advice; as a happy client is more likely to remain loyal to a salon, give it to them.
- Sort out any possible misunderstandings about ideas by using visuals. If you both agree on a bob, the client may be thinking of someone who works in her office. Words often mean different things to different people. Use magazines to prevent this happening, so both of you definitely know what you are agreeing to.

4.2 Design analysis

The simplest way of describing design analysis would be to say that it is an evaluation of the client, her hair and her needs, to determine how the hair should be styled to best enhance her appearance.

Design analysis is a detailed sequence of discrimination which eventually becomes second nature to the experienced stylist. It is not just a matter of creating a style which is suitable for the shape of the client's face because the total look also includes both lifestyle and manageability of the intended style. Ask your client how she manages her hair at home. Does she blow dry it or use heated rollers? How does she feel about her hair at this particular moment in time? What does she like or dislike about it? The client may be greatly influenced by partners or friends who might have suggested totally unsuitable styles. If this is the case, try to suggest alternatives (perhaps based on the client's original idea) backed up by ease of after-care or fashionability.

Never make a derogatory remark about a client to put a point across. We all know someone who would look better with an exceptionally long fringe, but we don't tell her! If a client resists your advice, it is ultimately her decision how her hair should look. You are responsible for carrying out the client's wishes, no matter how much you may disagree with the proposed idea. When considering the client, the design analysis can be broken down into different parts according to the client's needs. What follows, is a consideration of these parts.

Face shape in relation to hair design

Whatever the cutting or styling technique used, the one factor that never changes is the importance of creating a style to suit the shape of the face. We can isolate facial form into the seven principal shapes, illustrated in Fig. 4.1:

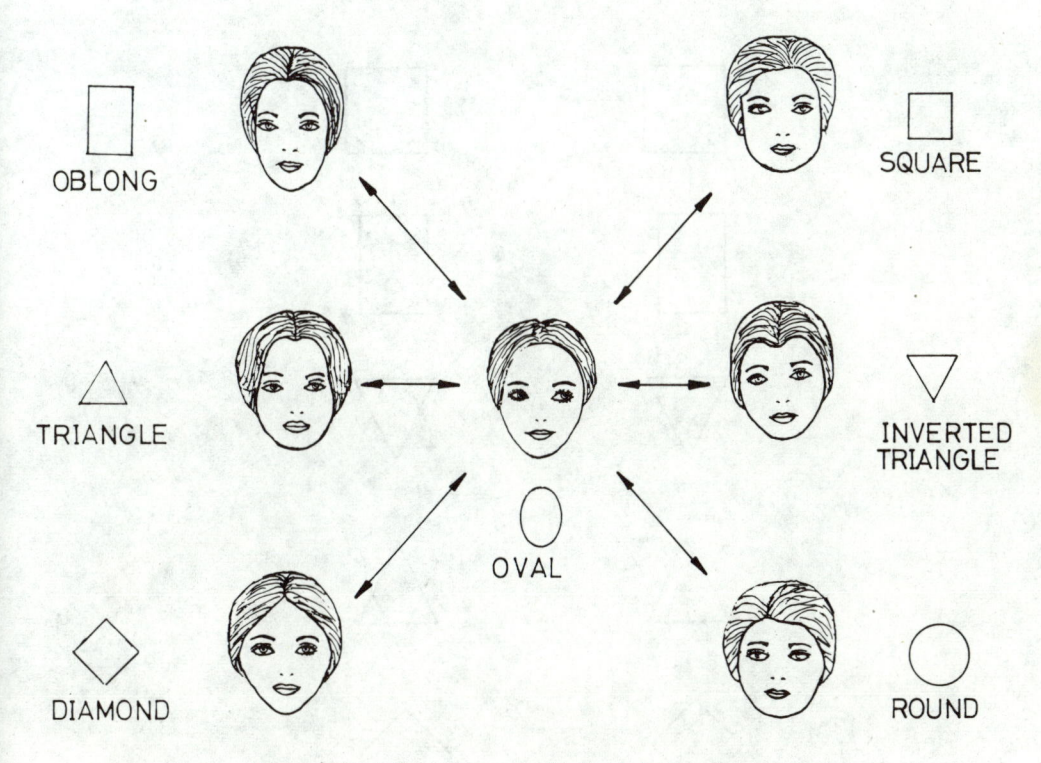

Fig. 4.1 The seven principal face shapes.

86 Cutting and Styling: a salon handbook

- Oval
- Oblong
- Square
- Triangular
- Inverted triangular (heart)
- Diamond
- Round

The oval face is considered as the ideal shape for which to design a hairstyle. This is because there are no irregular contours or proportions present which will need to be balanced or camouflaged by the hair design. Therefore, it can be said that when dealing with all of the other face

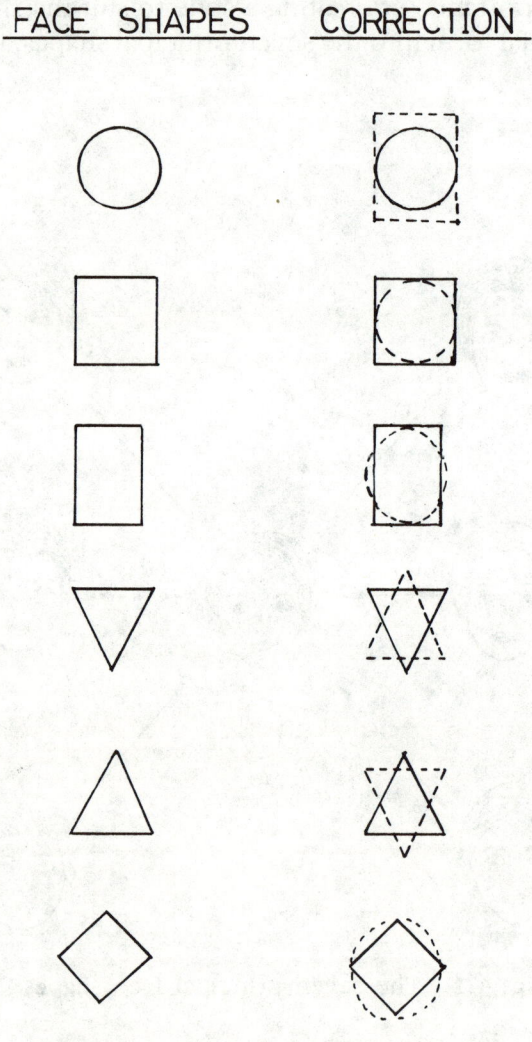

Fig. 4.2 Balancing face shapes.

shapes, we are aiming at creating the illusion of an oval face by the line and balance of the hair.

The principle of balancing facial shape can be seen in the series of diagrams in Fig. 4.2. We will now consider the styles that can be used under two headings: positive styles (styles that work to make the face shape appear oval) and negative styles (the styles that should be avoided as they do nothing, or make the shape even more prominent).

Positive styles	Negative styles
Round Styles which add height and are long and narrow through the sides.	Styles which accentuate the roundness of the face, such as tight perms, one-length cuts and round shapes.
Square Round shapes which soften the angular lines of the face.	Square cut bobs, geometric or angular shapes.
Oblong Asymmetrical shapes which widen the face and add interest.	Styles which are short at the sides and nape and are swept upwards to create height.
Inverted triangle or heart Styles which are full at the bottom to widen the chin and narrow through the top.	Styles which are high and wide through the cheek bone area, as these emphasise the narrow chin.
Triangular Shapes which are wide and full through the top and narrower through the sides. Longer hair will detract from any angular jawline.	Styles which are cut narrow through the top or very short styles as these both emphasise the wide jawline.
Diamond Round shapes which soften the angular lines of the face, which are narrow through the sides and mid-chin length to widen the chin.	Styles which are high, short or full at the sides as these will emphasise the narrow chin and wide cheek bones.

Body shape

Just as there is an ideal face shape there is also an ideal in body proportions. The height of a person should be seven or eight times the size of their head. If someone is short the hairstyle should be designed to give an illusion of extra height, while the opposite would be true for someone who is tall. The hairstyle should balance and harmonise with the height and build of the client. If the head of the client looks small design a style to make it look bigger; if it looks large design one to make it look smaller. Remember to take a look at clients while they are walking to gauge their exact height and the way they 'carry' themselves. There are no 'hard and fast' set rules about designing a style to suit body shape as face shape and facial features are so important in coming to the correct conclusion.

Head shape

Although our heads all consist of the same bones and conform to a recognisable 'skull' shape, there will be differences of form of some clients to be noted by the stylist. Feel the client's head with your hands. Are there any protrusions? Notable differences in head shape can be felt in the parietal and occipital areas (see Fig. 4.3). Some heads are either flatter or rounder here, and you may have to make adjustments in the style so the hair lies as you intend it to. You may also discover warts, cysts or scarring which were not evident from just combing the hair.

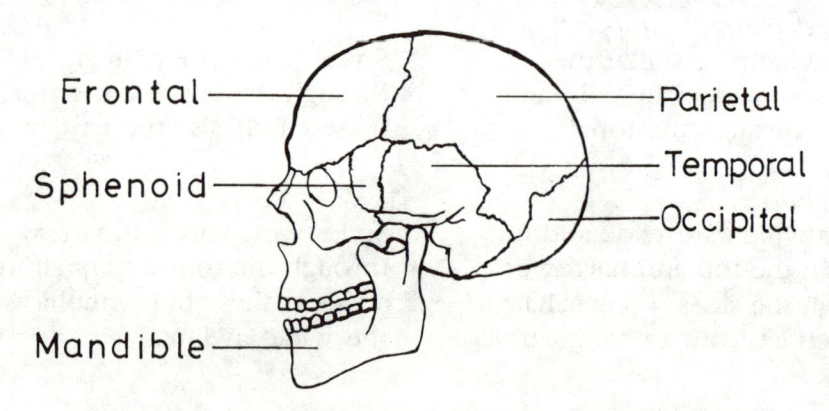

Fig. 4.3 The human skull, showing the main bones.

Facial features

Facial features include the eyes, nose and mouth. Styles can be designed which detract from or emphasise such facial features. An example of this is when a large prominent nose may be detracted from by dressing the front hair slightly at an angle, rather than symmetrically. Straight fringes will draw attention to wrinkled eyes whereas they will be softened by dressing the hair angled away from the face. A prominent profile will be accentuated by a style swept backwards off the face, so it is better to have the hair softly framing the face.

The neck
A long 'swan' neck will be accentuated if the hair is cut short or unswept at the nape, so the hair should be kept long to disguise the neck. Similarly, a short neck will be lengthened by cutting the hair short in the nape.

The ears
Protruding ears can be disguised by dressing the hair over them.

Hair density

Density is the term that describes the amount of hairs on a person's head, or more exactly, how closely spaced the hairs are. The more hairs per square centimetre or inch, the denser the hair is. Because of hair density, it may not always be possible to recreate certain styles on individual clients. Hair density may also differ on different areas of the same head. Actually put your fingers into the hair of the client to assess the density. Words used to describe density of hair include thick, medium, fine and sparse.

Hair texture

Hair texture refers to the thickness or diameter of individual hairs. It can be judged by taking individual hairs between the thumb and forefinger to feel whether they are fine, medium or thick. You will also be able to feel whether the hair is soft and pliable or coarse and hard. The term texture can also be used to describe how curly, wavy or straight the hair is and this should be considered for the suitability of particular hairstyles. For example, very curly hair would be difficult for the client to manage if it was cut into a square bob and stretched smooth by blow drying, as it would quickly revert back to being curly. Words used to describe texture include wiry, coarse, fine, pliable, frizzy, wavy, straight, hard, lank, etc.

Hair condition

The condition of the hair is important because the stylist should establish any previous chemical or physical damage that the hair has sustained. For example, highly bleached hair will have suffered from internal oxidation damage to the cortex, as well as external damage to the cuticle. It will be less elastic than hair in good condition and will therefore not hold a set or blow dry as well. Hair condition can be assessed by carrying out porosity and elasticity tests (these were fully described in both *Colouring – A Salon Handbook* and *Perming and Straightening – A Salon Handbook*). Words used to describe the condition of hair include dry, damaged, sensitised, split, oily, porous, dull, shiny, etc. For more detail on hair condition and conditioning treatments see Chapter 7.

Hair growth patterns

The direction of hair growth is very important because nothing a stylist can do will alter how the hair grows naturally. This means that forcing the hair in the opposite direction to its growth can often spell disaster because it will not lie properly and will fight to lie in its natural direction. This is particularly evident if a widow's peak is present on the front hairline, for example. A widow's peak is a strong, centre forward growing peak of hair found on the front hairline. Trying to style the hair into a full fringe would be difficult because it is going against the direction of the natural growth. The stylist may manage to make the hair look acceptable but the hair would soon separate and lift at the widow's peak and the client may find it very difficult to manage.

A cowlick is also found on the front hairline and is a strong growth of hair which grows in a sworl. Again, fighting the natural hair growth direction is not recommended. It is better to work with the natural lie of the hair.

The nape hairline will have its own unique pattern of growth. It may be low in the neck and grow to one side or be high and grow in the centre. The hair at the nape should not be forced against its natural growth or it may stick out the day after styling. It is not usually recommended to cut above the natural hairline because of this problem, but false hairlines can be created using scissors, razors, or clippers (see Chapter 5 – *Cutting*).

The crown is usually situated at the top or back of the head and forms the natural hair growth pattern for this area. Occasionally, two crowns may be detected, this being referred to as a double crown.

A natural parting is where the hair falls and parts naturally from the front hairline to the crown(s). To find out how to find a natural parting, see 4.6, Making partings.

The true lie of the hair can only properly be seen when the hair is wet because certain hair growth peculiarities may be disguised by the styling technique used previously by the client. The amount of lift at the roots of the hair can also more easily be seen when the hair is wet. Look for unusual root movements and hair growth direction. Words used to describe hair growth include cowlick, widow's peak, crown, natural parting, root lift, root direction, etc.

Lifestyle of a client

A client's lifestyle often determines the amount of time and money that they can afford to spend on their hair. A young, working mother will not be able to give a lot of time to her hair and so would want a style that is easily managed. Certain occupations such as nursing and the police place restrictions on individuals to conform to particular regulations for their hair. It may be that the hair must be worn up at work or that it should not touch the neck of a uniform.

The occasion

Although the majority of the stylist's work consists of everyday, wearable styles, clients often go to a salon for their hair to be styled for a special occasion. The best example is the bride who wants to have her hair different for her wedding day. In this instance, the stylist should see the client for several appointments before the 'big day' to work on different ideas which complement the head-dress, veil and outfit. Some salons actually set up a bride service which offers special rates if all the bridesmaids and some guests visit the salon. A stylist may visit the family home immediately prior to the wedding to attend to the head-dresses, veils, hair and make-up.

The client's age

Ultimately it is the bone structure of the client's face and head that determine the most suitable style. Modern styles can and should be worn by the older client, the difference being that hard lines should be softened and movement should be added to the style, as this is more flattering than very straight lines. Judge the age of your client – do not ask!

4.3 Design analysis — at a glance

Until design analysis becomes second nature, so that you do it unconsciously, use these guidelines. Tick the appropriate boxes and enter any necessary details. You may find that the quality of the hair, things like texture and condition, falls in more than one category. Keep this list well away from the client!

Face shape
Oval ☐ Oblong ☐ Square ☐ Triangular ☐
Inverted triangular ☐ Diamond ☐ Round ☐

Body shape
Tall and lean ☐ Short and fat ☐ The ideal ☐
Short upper body with slim waist ☐
Slim upper body with heavy thighs ☐

Head shape
Scars ☐ Cysts ☐ Warts ☐
Details of protrusions in occipital and parietal area..............................

Facial features
Features to emphasise..
Features to detract...

The neck
Long and slim ☐ Short and fat ☐ Long and broad ☐
Short and slim ☐ Average ☐

The ears
Degree of protrusion...
Size: average ☐ large ☐ small ☐

Hair density
Thick ☐ Average ☐ Thin ☐ Sparse ☐
Details of any baldness/thinning..

Hair texture
Coarse ☐ Wiry ☐ Frizzy ☐ Hard ☐
Pliable ☐ Soft ☐ Wavy ☐ Straight ☐
Curly ☐ Lank ☐ Fine ☐ Other..............................

Hair condition
Damaged ☐ Split ☐ Porous ☐ Sensitive ☐
Dull ☐ Dry ☐ Shiny ☐ Oily ☐

Hair growth patterns
Cowlick ☐ Widow's peak ☐ Crown ☐ Double crown ☐
Details of front hairline..
Details of nape hairline...
Details of root lift and growth direction...
Details of natural parting..

Client's lifestyle
Weekly visits to the salon ☐
Regular (between 4 and 8 weeks) visits to the salon ☐
Details of restrictions to style..

Occasion
Everyday style ☐
Details of special occasion...

Client's age
Under 5 ☐ 5–13 ☐ 13–16 ☐ 16–20 ☐ 20–25 ☐
25–35 ☐ 35–45 ☐ 45–55 ☐ 55–65 ☐ over 65 ☐

4.4 Preparation

Gowning a client

Why should a client wear a gown?
A client's clothes must be adequately protected by a gown from both hair clippings and products. If a client's clothing is spoilt, they are within their rights to sue the salon. If hair clippings get inside a client's clothing, she will be itching for hours afterwards, and not thinking very kindly of the salon!

Every client should have a freshly laundered gown. If this is not possible, no part of the gown should come into direct contact with the client's skin; a neck strip of disposable crepe paper should be placed between the client's neck and the gown.

Gowns should be made of cotton or a mixture containing some cotton (polyester and cotton, etc.), as this will be more comfortable for the client to wear, especially in hot weather. Gowns can either be tied at the neck or be the wrap-over type with a tie belt at the waist. Whichever type is used, gowns should be large enough to cover the client's clothing adequately and should not be tied too tightly.

When should a plastic cape be put on a client?
Plastic capes are used in many salons when perming, colouring or cutting, as an added protection. They are put on over the gown and are secured at the neck. Always make sure that jewellery and clothing (such as high-necked sweaters) are not causing an obstruction. Politely ask your client to remove such items if they might be damaged, or if they could hinder you while working on the client. Be careful not to get the gown caught on a jewellery clasp; there are few sights as embarrassing as beads from a necklace falling about all over the floor!

Combing and brushing the hair before a service

The hair should be combed and then brushed during the intitial discussion that takes place between the stylist and the client at the beginning of the appointment. However, the hair should only be combed and not brushed before a chemical treatment such as perming or tinting. This is because brushing could scratch and irritate the scalp.

Why should the hair be combed and brushed before a service?
Combing and brushing the hair makes it easier to work with and more comfortable for the client. It frees the hair from tangles, previous

backcombing, dust, dirt and scaling, and loosens hairspray. You can also check the scalp for lice and nits without the client being aware.

How should the hair be combed?
Using a wide-toothed comb, begin in the nape region at the points of the hair, gradually working upwards towards the scalp. The hand not holding the comb should be positioned as shown in Fig. 4.4, to support the head. The comb should be held upright, not flattened which would scratch the head, and drawn through the hair without pulling or tugging. As each mesh of hair is combed, another mesh of hair is taken and the same procedure is followed, working over the entire head. Hair should not be combed starting at the roots because the tangles will be pushed down to the points. If this happens the tangles are difficult to remove and will cause discomfort for the client.

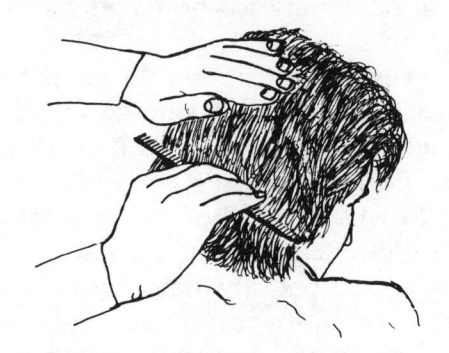

Fig. 4.4 Combing hair, one hand supporting head.

Why should the hair be brushed?
Hair is brushed before a service for the following reasons:

- to relax and soothe the client;
- to remove loose hair and debris;
- to stimulate the blood supply to the scalp.

N.B. Wet hair should never be brushed to remove tangles as this causes over-stretching and subsequent breakage.

How should the hair be brushed?
After combing, the hair can be brushed using either single or double brushing, as illustrated in Fig. 4.5.
Single brushing. Using one hand to support the head, the hair is brushed beginning at the hair points at the nape, gradually brushing closer to the scalp. This is continued over the whole head in a smoothing, stroking action.
Double brushing. As the name implies, double brushing is carried out using two hairbrushes. The brushes are used in a rolling action with one of the brushes always in contact with the hair. As one of the brushes leaves the hair, the other hand rolls over the first in a smooth, consistent pattern of movement. This type of brushing usually precedes a hair treatment (see Chapter 7).

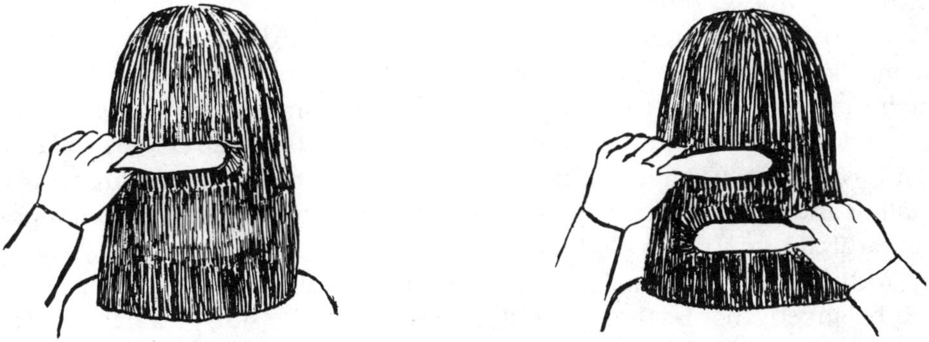

Fig. 4.5 Single and double brushing.

4.5 Shampooing

For many of the hairdressing services offered in a salon the hair is shampooed. Shampoo is a Hindu word, which means 'to clean'. It is important that the shampooing does not cause any discomfort or irritation for the client. A good shampoo will soothe and relax the client, making her visit more enjoyable and the stylist's job easier. Dealing with a client who has just been soaked at the basin is not easy, and should *never* happen!

What are the reasons for shampooing hair?
Hair is shampooed for two main reasons:

(a) to cleanse the hair and scalp by removing dirt, scales of keratin, stale perspiration, grease and other debris such as hairspray or oil-based dressing products; and
(b) to prepare the hair for subsequent hairdressing processes (shampooed hair absorbs more moisture than hair that is simply wetted with water).

If the hair is not properly cleansed, grease and dirt may interfere with the absorption of products by the hair. It will be impossible to achieve body and bounce with hair that is greasy. Clean hair is also less likely to be a breeding ground for bacteria and fungi. Although the primary purpose of shampooing is to clean the hair, special shampoos are available to aid certain hair and scalp conditions. The shampoo that you use must be selected with the particular client and hairdressing service in mind. For example, if you were preparing a client for a chemical treatment, you would not use a shampoo with any special ingredients that might produce a barrier on the hair.

96 Cutting and Styling: a salon handbook

Soap or soapless shampoos?
Shampoos today contain soapless detergents that do not react with hard water like the older soap shampoos. A soap shampoo reacts with the calcium in hard water to form insoluble soap scum (the sodium stearate in the soap forms the scum, calcium stearate, once the soap begins to lather) so it is of no real use in the modern salon. Furthermore, soap shampoos are alkaline and make the cuticle of the hair swell, whereas soapless shampoos are naturally neutral or slightly alkaline but can easily be made acidic by the addition of suitable acids (citric acid, for example). Many shampoos are acid-balanced; that is, they have the same pH as the skin and hair (a pH of between 4.5 and 5.5). Soapless shampoos can degrease the hair too much if they are too strong, as well as having a greater tendency to produce dermatitis in the hairdresser's hands or on the client's scalp. These two drawbacks are fully accepted by the industry, and it is important to take suitable precautions. (See *Hygiene – A Salon Handbook*.)

How do shampoos clean hair?

We say that shampoos contain detergents. The selected detergent must not be too alkaline as this will roughen the hair, nor must it damage the eyes or irritate the scalp too much. Shampoos must also produce a good lather as it is the lather that keeps the detergent in close contact with the skin and hair, enabling it to be clearly seen where the shampoo has been applied.

Actual detergency depends on the detergent molecule having both a hydrophilic (water-loving) and hydrophobic (water-hating) group of atoms. These are usually arranged into a hydrophilic head (which may have a positive or negative charge, or no charge at all) and a hydrophobic tail (consisting of a chain of carbon and hydrogen atoms). Such a molecule of detergent is illustrated in Fig. 4.6. If it is at an interface (the point where air and water meet, such as at the surface of water in a glass) the hydrophilic head will be attracted to the water while the hydrophobic tail will stick out into the air. The detergent will form a single layer on the water surface. With grease and water, such as would be found on a dirty hair, the hydrophilic heads stick out into water while the hydrophobic tails are attracted by the grease. Although these two facts may not explain too much to you straight away, Figs. 4.7 and 4.8 should do.

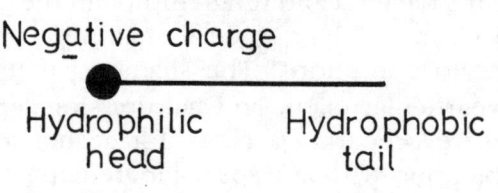

Fig. 4.6 A molecule of detergent.

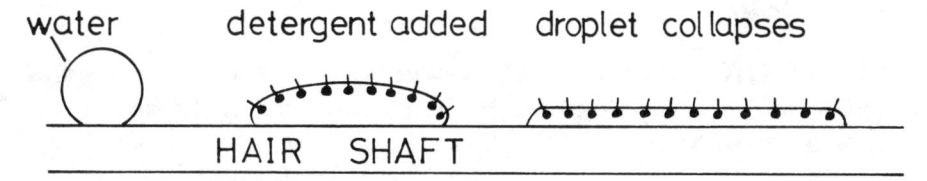

Fig. 4.7 How a detergent improves the wetting of hair by reducing the surface tension of water.

In Fig. 4.7 a droplet of water has been dropped onto a hair. Because of surface tension, an inward pulling force that is exerted at the outer surface of liquids, it stays as a rounded globule. As soon as some detergent is added the hydrophilic heads break this surface tension and the water droplet flattens out. The detergent, being a surface active agent (often shortened to the word surfactant), has lowered the surface tension of water. This is important because it means that the detergent allows hair to be wetted better than by water alone.

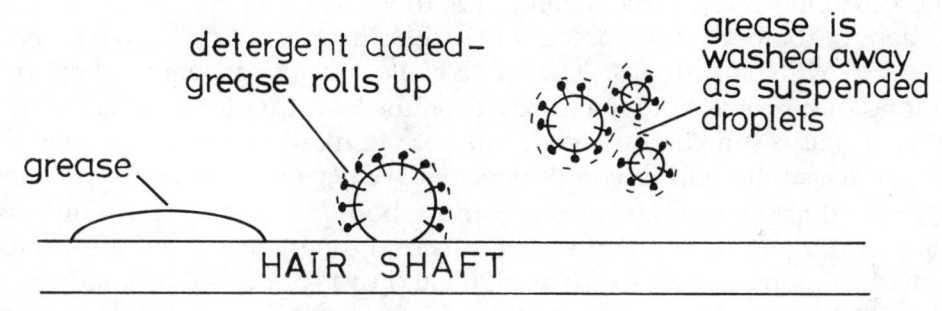

Fig. 4.8 How a detergent removes grease from the hair during shampooing.

In Fig, 4.8, a globule of grease is present on the hair. As it is attracted to the hair it is flattened out onto the hair surface. Once detergent is applied to the hair the hydrophilic tails penetrate the surface of the grease and the negatively charged heads cause it to roll up into a globule. This gives the grease less surface contact with the hair, until eventually it is suspended in the water to form an emulsion (oil droplets suspended in water) which can easily be removed as the hair is rinsed. Thus a detergent is also an emulsifying agent.

Emulsions are mixtures of oil and water. Normally oil would float on the surface of water and would not mix for very long if shaken together. Because the detergent, as an emulsifying agent, is partially soluble in both oil and water, it forms a bridge between the two and stops them from separating out into two layers again.

Special shampoos

Although we have said that soapless shampoos are the industry standard, the actual detergent and extra ingredients can vary in the shampoos for different types of hair:

Greasy hair

The actual percentage of soapless detergent in a shampoo for greasy hair varies from the usual 15–20 per cent to as high as 50 per cent of the shampoo. This means that the shampoo will remove the grease more quickly; but it does nothing to *prevent* greasy hair. Lemon shampoo is often mentioned as being a shampoo for greasy hair, but lemon does nothing to remove the grease. Therefore, if you want value for money, shampoos for greasy hair do contain more detergent! A shampoo for greasy hair will contain few oily or fatty substances, which would be found in shampoos for normal or dry hair.

Dry hair

These shampoos are of two main types, those which degrease the hair less because of their reduced content of soapless detergent (about 10 per cent) or those with added oils. The added oils include coconut, olive and almond oils, residues of which are left on the hair. Lanolin (natural sheep's sebum) is also sometimes added, but bear in mind that some people are allergic to lanolin. Other conditioners such as egg or beer are sometimes added and claimed to give the hair more body, but are in truth, quickly rinsed from the hair when used as shampoo ingredients and are pretty ineffective. One egg added to a 1000 gallon vat of normal shampoo will still make it an egg shampoo! Beware of herb shampoos as well; herb extracts do little for a shampoo except possibly to scent it!

Dandruff

Anti-dandruff shampoos contain substances which claim to reduce the multiplication of the epidermal cells, and thus reduce subsequent scaling. There are two main active ingredients found in such shampoos, but zinc pyrithione (also called zinc omadine) is by far the most popular of the two. It has a concentration of between 2–3 per cent in a soapless detergent base and also has antiseptic properties. Those shampoos containing the other ingredient, selenium sulphide, are rare now because so many people are allergic to sulphur. This type of shampoo would contain between 2–5 per cent selenium sulphide and should be asked for in the chemist. Someone with dry hair may find it beneficial to use a sulphur shampoo as it stimulates the sebaceous glands, this being the reason for the popularity of such shampoos with sailors who tend to suffer from dry hair because of their work.

Design Analysis and Preparation

Damaged hair
If the hair has a porous cuticle and structural damage such as split ends, protein shampoos can be very beneficial. The shampoos contain broken down protein (often labelled as hydrolysed protein) in the form of short chains of amino acids. These are substantive to hair; that is, they cling to it, filling in some of the damaged areas and making split ends cling together. Any such repairs achieved are temporary, however, and there is no permanent change.

Psoriasis
If a client has psoriasis the use of a coal tar shampoo may be beneficial as it can reduce scaling.

Coloured hair
Once hair begins to fade there are colour shampoos available to revive it. These range from camomile for blonde hair, henna for red highlights, walnut for brown hair to a range of temporary and semi-permanent dyes in shampoo bases. Peroxide, of 10 volume (3 per cent) strength, is often added to shampoo as a brightener for light brown or blonde hair.

Itchy scalps
Clients with itchy scalps are likely to scratch them and cause subsequent infections. They should be encouraged to use a medicated shampoo. These can be of two types, cationic or with added antiseptics. Cationic shampoos have a positive charge which is attracted to the overall negative charge of hair. Most other shampoos are anionic, that is, they have a negative charge. The cationic detergent used is usually cetrimide which coats the hair, leaving an antiseptic film behind. It does not lather very well and can damage the eyes (use a backwash as protection against this as cetrimide can cause the transparent cornea in front of the eye lens to become opaque), but can be a useful shampoo. Other shampoos contain an anionic detergent together with an antiseptic such as hexachlorophene or resorcinol.

After alkaline treatments
The shampoo to be used should neutralise any excess alkalinity and close the cuticle, so must be acid. The preferred acidity is similar to that of the skin and hair (a pH of 4.5–5.5; hence the term 'acid-balanced'). Such shampoos will help tinted hair resist fading because of the closed cuticle.

Are baby shampoos milder than normal shampoos?
No! Baby shampoos are formulated with a different soapless detergent so that they do not irritate the eyes. They are no better for frequent hair washing, though many hairdressers tell their clients this...

100 Cutting and Styling: a salon handbook

Do thick shampoos clean hair better than thin ones?
If you were given the choice of a thick shampoo or a thin runny one, it is likely that you would prefer the thick one. In use both should clean the hair equally well, but you might be tempted to use words like 'richer' to describe the thick shampoo. The creamy shampoo is in fact only a thin shampoo which has been thickened. The manufacturers often use common salt (sodium chloride) to thicken their shampoos. You could try this yourself by slowly adding salt to some shampoo and stirring. It will continue to thicken for some time and will then suddenly become thin again, as an excess of salt reverses the thickening process. Other chemicals are also used to thicken shampoos, parabens being a group of chemicals used to thicken many hairdressing products.

What should be the client's position during shampooing?

The best position for a client having a shampoo is in a reclined position at a backwash basin, as illustrated in Fig. 4.9. Because the client is leaning backwards the face remains dry and the risk of anything entering the eyes is drastically reduced. Forward wash basins are becoming must less popular as even with a cloth over the eyes the face still usually gets wet, possibly ruining make-up.

Place a towel around the client's shoulders, tucking it into the collar of the gown. The client should then be comfortably seated; you may have to adjust either the chair or basin height so that the neck rests in the central neck-rest of the basin. You can either stand alongside or behind your client.

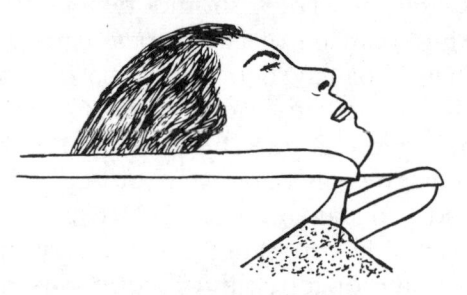

Fig. 4.9 Backwash.

How is a shampoo carried out?

(1) Select the appropriate shampoo according to the condition of the hair and the scalp.
(2) Turn on the cold water tap first and gradually add the hot water until you have created a comfortable temperature. Test this on either the back of your hand or the inside of your wrist.
(3) Shield the client's face from any splashes by placing your hand on the hairline as shown in Fig. 4.10. The palm of your hand should always be facing the jet of water and is moved to whichever part of the front

hairline needs protection. Always check with your client that the water temperature is comfortable. If it needs readjusting move the water spray away from the client's head. Hold the water spray near the client's head to avoid unnecessary splashing and turn off the water once you have thoroughly wetted the hair.

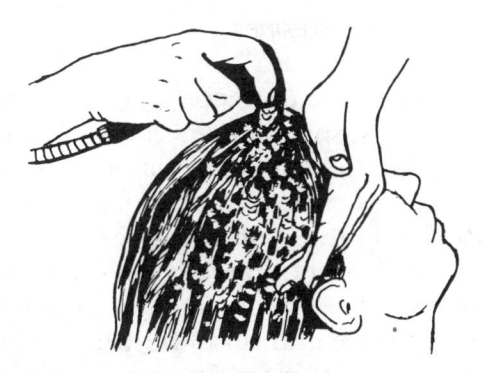

Fig. 4.10 Washing the hair.

(4) Pour the shampoo into the palm of your hand. Spread it between your hands and smooth it through the hair to distribute it evenly. Don't put the shampoo directly onto one area of the head, or it will not spread out evenly; it would also feel cold to the client and might cause dermatitis where it was applied because of its concentration in one area. You are better to apply too little shampoo, rather than too much as it is easy to apply more. Having your shampoo in pump dispenser bottles will make it last longer and encourage good application techniques.

(5) Begin your massage making sure that your nails do not scratch the scalp. The pressure of your fingers should be adjusted according to particular clients so that they find it comfortable (this varies from client to client). Using the pads of your fingers, massage the scalp in circular movements, ensuring that the whole head is covered. A common complaint from clients is that the nape area is missed.

(6) Turn on the water as before until the correct temperature is reached, then thoroughly rinse the hair.

(7) Apply more shampoo (less than on the first wash) and repeat the massage and rinse. The hair should now be 'squeaky' clean, because all the oil has been removed. Running your hands through the clients hair will confirm this for you.

(8) Press excessive water out of the scalp using your hands in firm, stroking movements from hairline to nape.

(9) Wrap a clean dry towel over the client's head to prevent drips and gently raise the client into an upright position. The shampoo should have been so relaxing for the client that she should be disappointed it is all over!

(10) Seat your client at a styling unit and gently towel-dry the hair.

(11) Using a wide-toothed comb, disentangle the hair and comb it straight back from the face. Change the towel around the client's shoulders if this became wet during the shampoo.

Shampoo guidelines

- Select the correct shampoo for each client.
- Use freshly laundered towels for each client.
- Give the client your individual attention.
- Check water temperature before wetting the client's hair.
- Apply the shampoo over the whole head by applying to your hands first and not directly onto the client's head.
- Check the pressure of your massage with the client.
- Massage and rinse the whole head thoroughly.
- Hold the water spray close to the head to avoid splashing.
- Always replace a wet towel with a dry one to ensure client comfort.
- *If the client really likes the shampoo that you use, sell her a bottle!*

4.6 Making partings

There are no rules about making partings in hair; they can be any length, at any angle and at any place on the head. Partings can be straight, curved, slanted, zig-zag, high, low, centre or side. The purpose of a parting is to assist in creating an illusory effect in hair design, as follows:

(a) Straight partings from the forehead to the crown will add length to the face.

(b) Short partings increase the height of the head and the style.

(c) The greater the angle of the parting, the wider the head will appear.

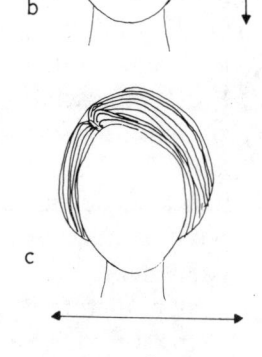

Fig. 4.11

Finding the natural parting

A natural parting can only be found when the hair is wet. After disentangling, comb the hair back straight from the face using the wide teeth of your comb. Keep the hair combed close to the head and then place your other hand on the head and gently nudge the hair forward. The hair will then break to reveal the natural parting.

Although it is usually recommended to use the natural parting, it is sometimes necessary to make your own parting elsewhere. Working against the natural parting is useful for obtaining height in some styles and the clever placing of a parting can cause thin faces to appear broader and wide faces to look narrower. Many men with thinning heads of hair assume that having a low side parting will make them appear to have more hair. When making a parting, to balance the comb, place you index finger on top of the comb.

4.7 Questions

1. What is the 'total look'?
2. Why should the client never be taken straight through to have her hair washed?
3. What are the reasons for consultation at the beginning of the appointment?
4. What do you understand by the term 'design analysis'?
5. List, with simple diagrams, the seven main face shapes.
6. In the form of a table, list positive styles for these shapes.
7. In the form of a table, list negative styles for these shapes.
8. How does body shape influence the selected style?
9. Give examples of how you would take the emphasis away from prominent facial features.
10. How would you disguise prominent ears?
11. What is hair density?
12. How can hair texture influence the selected style?
13. How do you check the internal and external condition of hair?
14. Why are hair growth patterns important considerations?
15. With reasons, should the growth pattern be checked on wet or on dry hair?
16. What type of service could the salon provide for a wedding?
17. How does the age of the client influence the selected style?
18. Why should a client wear a gown?

19 If you cannot provide each client with a fresh gown, what hygienic precaution should be taken?
20 Why should the hair be combed and brushed before a treatment?
21 How should the hair be combed?
22 Why should wet hair never be brushed to remove tangles?
23 What are the two main reasons for shampooing hair?
24 Would you use soap or soapless shampoos in the salon?
25 What is the disadvantage of an alkaline shampoo?
26 How is scum formed with soap and hard water?
27 What do the terms 'hydrophobic' and 'hydrophilic' mean?
28 How does a detergent act at the interface between water and air?
29 How does a detergent act at the interface between oil and water?
30 What is a surfactant?
31 Why do we say that a detergent is an emulsifying agent?
32 Describe the difference between shampoos for greasy, dry and damaged hair?
33 What shampoos would you use on a client who had either dandruff or psoriasis?
34 Why might special shampoos be used on coloured hair?
35 Are baby shampoos more suitable for frequent washing of hair than normal shampoos?
36 Does a thick shampoo clean hair better than a thin one?
37 How should a client be positioned during shampooing?
38 Why should cold water be turned on first?
39 How do you shield the client's eyes from water and chemicals?
40 How and why should a shampoo be applied?
41 When massaging clients, why should you check your finger pressure with them?
42 How would you remove excessive water from the hair?
43 What use have partings when creating a hairstyle?

5
Cutting

There is more to cutting hair than simply reducing its length. It takes technical skill, care and imagination to produce good results as every head is different and presents its own problems.

Just as a sculptor chips and carves a shape into marble or wood, the hairdresser can carefully remove the unwanted hair with the same degree of precision. A good haircut is the basis of a manageable style and is usually a high priority when clients choose a salon or stylist. It is often the case that young hairdressers fail to recognise the importance of being able to perform a particular haircut even though it is currently not in fashion. A competent stylist is equipped with *all* the cutting skills and carefully chooses the appropriate techniques to achieve the desired style. Many styles can be accomplished only by incorporating several techniques on the same head, with sometimes enormous variations. An experienced stylist can look at a head of hair and identify what cutting methods were used to achieve it. This is a particularly valuable skill when a client brings a picture with her to the salon for the stylist to copy.

It is impossible to learn how to cut hair from just reading a book because it is not like painting by numbers. As we have already said, every head is different and so poses its own unique problems. It is practical experience that makes the hairdresser a good cutter, combined with a dedicated attitude to produce a high standard of work. For these reasons, this chapter will be concerned with the principles and concepts of haircutting aided by some step-by-step photographs of styles created by master craftsmen of the industry.

5.1 Introduction to cutting methods

Scissors can be used on wet or dry hair. Basically, there are three cutting methods that can be carried out, using different scissor techniques as well as razors or clippers. They are:

(1) one length;
(2) graduation;
(3) layer.

(1) One length

A one length haircut would be described as the hair being cut to fall to the same outside length. The weight and fullness of the haircut is around the perimeter of the shape, while the inside hair has no shape or movement. For this reason (weight distribution), a one length haircut could be interpreted as having a slightly triangular appearance, due to the fullness achieved by the hair points ending at the same level, as shown in Fig. 5.1.

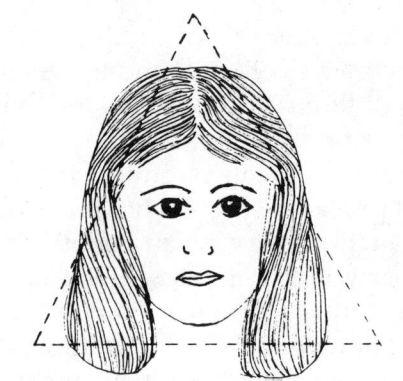

Fig. 5.1 One length cut.

(2) Graduation

A graduated haircut is different from a one length shape because the hair is held and cut at a specific angle to produce fullness blending into shorter lengths of hair. The weight and fullness of a graduated haircut moves up from the perimeter to a higher point and so has a slightly diamond shape, as shown in Fig. 5.2.

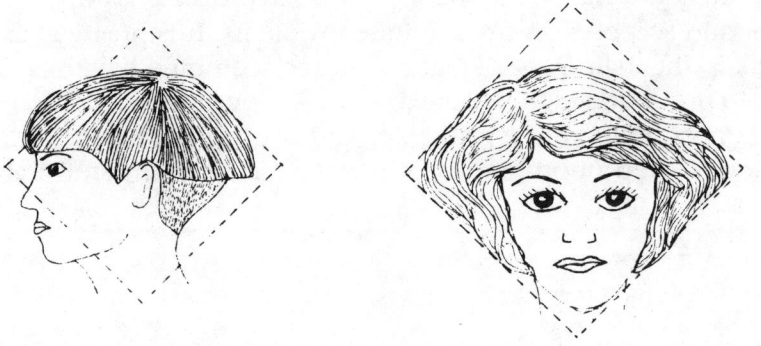

Fig. 5.2 Graduated cut.

(3) Layer

Layering reduces the hair length by holding and cutting the hair at an angle of 90 degrees to the shape of the head. The weight and fullness is evenly distributed, giving a round appearance to the style, as shown in Fig. 5.3.

It is not unusual to use more than one cutting method on a single head. Try looking at some style plates in trade magazines and see if you can work out how each was cut.

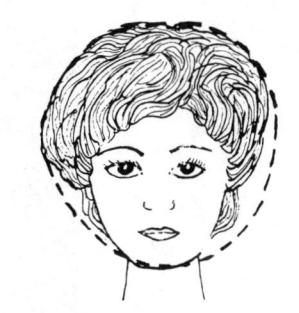

Fig. 5.3 Layer cut.

5.2 Introduction to scissor techniques

Scissors can be used in two main ways to achieve different effects. Again, more than one of these scissor techniques could be incorporated into a haircut to create the desired look:

(1) blunt or club cutting;
(2) tapering.

(1) Blunt or club cutting

Blunt or club cutting is the term used to describe the action of using scissors to remove hair by a straight cut, as shown in Fig. 5.4. (The same technique is demonstrated with clippers in Fig. 5.5.) This technique leaves the ends of the hair blunt and evenly finished at the same length. Club cutting is an ideal technique for cutting fine hair because it helps the hair

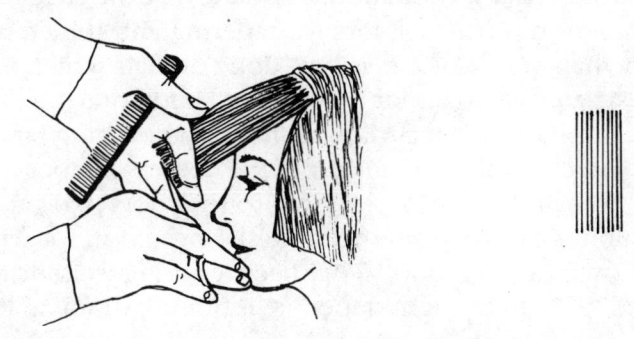

Fig. 5.4 Blunt or club cutting using scissors and the result on the hair.

feel and look heavier. Club cut hair is more difficult to backcomb and decreases the hair's natural tendency to curl.

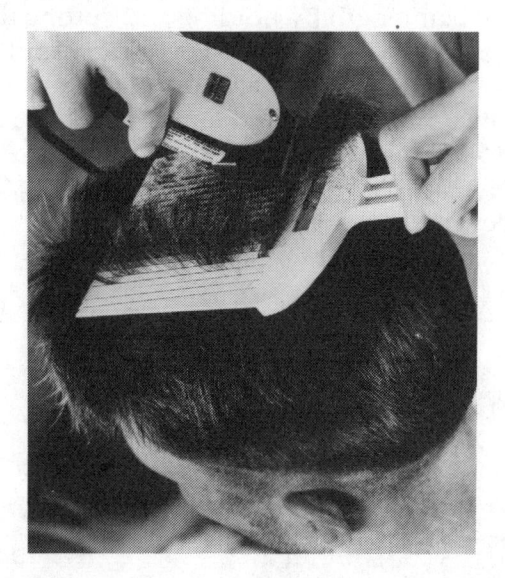

Fig. 5.5 Club cutting with clippers. In this case a special comb called the Brian Drumm Flattopper is used to lift the hair up. The resultant cut produces a level style on the crown which is very effective on Afro hair. (Courtesy of Brian Drumm.)

(2) Tapering

Tapering with scissors is also known as slithering or feathering. The scissors are used in a sliding action, backwards and forwards along the hair length. The scissors are allowed to open and close only slightly, using the heel of the scissors to cut the hair when the scissors are moving towards the head. Unlike club cutting, tapering has a thinning effect on the hair, creating shorter lengths which make tapered hair much easier to backcomb and increasing the natural tendency of the hair to curl. Figure 5.6 shows the action of the scissors for tapering and the effect produced.

Tapering the hair with scissors is best done on hair which is dry because the hair tends to cling together when wet, impairing the action of the scissors. A variation on this technique is the backcombing taper technique. The amount of backcombing determines the degree of taper to the mesh of hair because the hair pushed back down to the roots (backcombed) is not cut. The remaining hair is cut in the same sliding action for tapering as was previously shown in Fig. 5.6. The backcombing scissor technique is shown in Fig. 5.7. If a slight taper is required, then a lot of hair is backcombed.

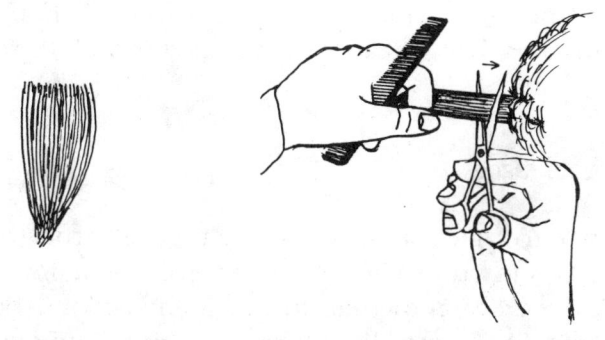

Fig. 5.6 Taper cutting scissors and the result.

Scissors can be used to taper wet hair like a razor, but only if they have a plain straight cutting edge (not serrated) and are very sharp. The mesh of hair is held and the open scissor blade is gently stroked towards the points. An open scissor blade used in this manner, or a razor, is never used in an upward direction (i.e. towards the scalp) because it would be in the opposite lie of the cuticle and would therefore cause uncomfortable pulling for the client and damage to the hair shaft.

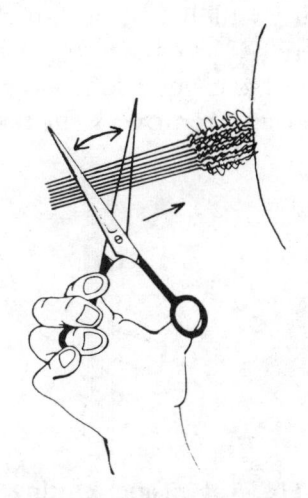

Fig. 5.7 Backcomb taper cutting technique.

5.3 Introduction to razor techniques

Razors should only be used on wet hair. Razor cutting dry hair would be painful for the client and bad for the razor. While razor cutting, both hands should move in unison. The hand holding the mesh of hair moves away as the blade approaches – an important movement to remember to avoid cutting the fingers! The blade is always moved towards you, never against the lie of the cuticle towards the scalp. Therefore, the stylist needs frequently to change position so that the correct angles of holding and cutting are maintained. In razor cutting it is the angle at which the blade is introduced to the hair and the amount of pressure used that determines the degree of taper and how much hair is removed. Although a razor is primarily used to taper hair, it can be used equally well to remove length and club cut the hair.

Taper cutting with a razor

When using a razor to taper cut, it is placed either underneath or above the mesh to be cut, as shown in Fig. 5.8(a) and (b). The hair is held and the razor blade is stroked down the hair in a scraping action from the middle lengths to the ends. For a very slight taper, use only minimum pressure or too much hair will be removed. Remember that it is the angle of the blade in relation to the mesh of hair that determines the amount of taper. If the razor is held with the back of the blade resting on the hair, the taper will be long and thin. Be careful not to overdo this as it may result in long wispy ends which will be difficult to manage. After taper cutting with a razor it may be necessary to cut the ends with scissors to remove any wispy ends that have been left. Don't make the mistake of cutting too far down the hair and remove your tapering.

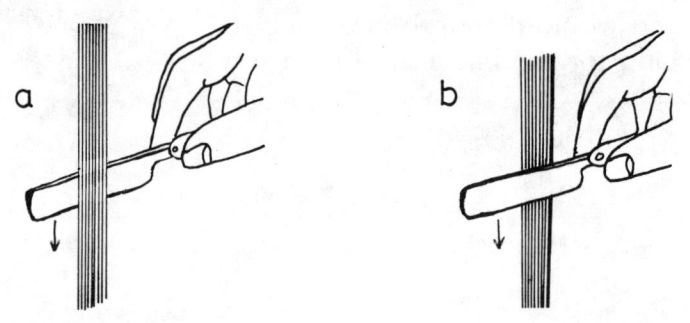

Fig. 5.8 Taper cutting with a razor (a) underneath a mesh of hair and (b) above a mesh of hair.

Club cutting with a razor

Unlike taper cutting with a razor, the blade is held at a right angle towards the mesh, as illustrated in Fig. 5.9. The mesh must be held taut so that the blade edge can slice through to achieve a clubbed cut. The actual cut is made between the fingers and the head, not directly over the fingers, using the same angles and positions of the hair as for club cutting using scissors.

Fig. 5.9 Club cutting with a razor, held at a 90° angle to the mesh of hair.

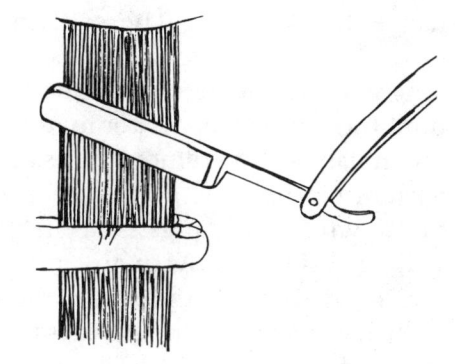

5.4 Methods of thinning hair

Thinning is the term given to cutting techniques which remove bulk and weight without affecting the overall length of the hair.

Thinning with notched blade scissors

Conventional scissors or razors can be used to remove excess bulk and weight from hair, although there are special thinning scissors available with notched teeth instead of blades. Thinning scissors are also called aescalops and can have one or both blades notched. Double-notched scissors remove *less* hair than thinning scissors with one notched and one plain blade. This can be seen in Fig. 5.10 which shows a magnified view of the two types of thinning scissors.

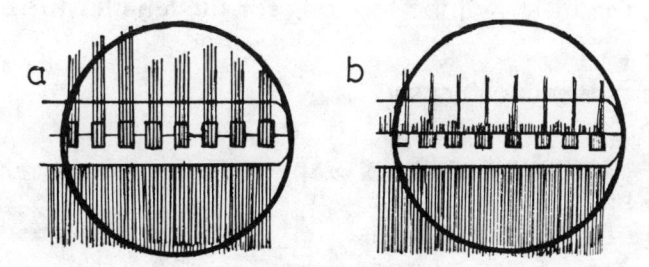

Fig. 5.10 The amount of hair cut with (a) double notch and (b) single notch thinning scissors.

Thinning scissors should be used on dry hair and are held in the same way as conventional haircutting scissors (i.e. with the thumb and third finger). A mesh of hair is held between the fingers, and the scissors are closed across the mesh at a distance of at least 4 cms (1½ inches) from the scalp to prevent spiky hairs from sticking through the top layers when the hair is combed flat. The scissors are closed once and then opened and moved down another 2–3 cms (1 inch) and a cut is made again. If the hair is long you may need to continue this movement down the length of the hair until the excess bulk is removed, but few cuts should be made or else too much hair will be removed. Use the closely set teeth of your cutting comb to remove the cut hair from the mesh while thinning as it helps you to estimate how many times you need to close the scissors on each mesh. The thinning scissors should be held straight across the mesh as shown in Fig. 5.11. Avoid using thinning scissors in the following areas:

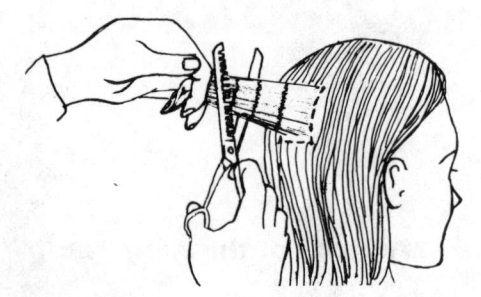

Fig. 5.11 Reducing bulk in hair using thinning scissors.

- closer than 4 cms to the scalp;
- on hairlines;
- at the crown;
- along partings.

Do not assume that you will need to thin the whole of the head. Use your fingers to test the bulk of the hair by pushing your hands into the hair and feeling it. If you plan to thin the hair all over the head, begin at the nape by taking vertical sections 1 cm wide and 5 cms long. If you take sections wider than 1 cm, the hair will pull when the scissors close. If they are too long, the mesh will be too long for the length of the blades.

Thinning with conventional scissors

The tapering technique can be used to thin hair by tapering the middle third of the mesh. This is shown in Fig. 5.12. Long, sweeping strokes are used, almost as though you are using the scissors to backcomb the hair.

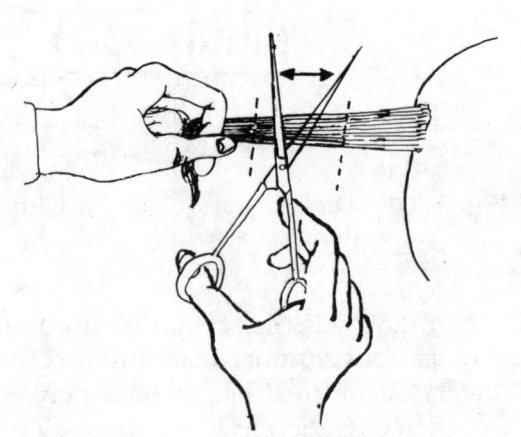

Fig. 5.12 Thinning hair using conventional scissors.

Thinning with a razor

Razors are only used on wet hair because razor cutting dry hair would quickly blunt the razor and be painful for the client. To remove excess bulk from hair using a razor, the tapering technique is used. To ensure that the overall length of the hair is not altered, use minimum pressure on the mesh and hold the blade so that the back rests on the hair, stroking the blade towards you.

5.5 Methods of texturising hair

Texturising is thinning the hair with the intention of creating visible short and long lengths of hair in a style and to add lift and support at the hair roots.

Texturising techniques using conventional scissors

There are many techniques which can be used to texturise hair and to achieve interesting differences in hair length in a style. Unlike thinning, texturising is intended to show visible variations between the hair lengths. You might know some of the techniques described here by different names. We have chosen four techniques which are widely used:

(1) weave cutting;
(2) chipping;
(3) channel cutting;
(4) pointing.

(1) Weave cutting

Weave cutting is used to reduce bulk, creating uneven hair lengths and giving a stranded effect. This is a particularly useful technique for styles which need to be spiky or stranded and full. It works on the principle that the hair which is woven out is cut shorter, thus helping to push up and support the longer lengths. The actual weaving is done using the closed blades of the scissors, as shown in Fig. 5.13, the same way as in weave colouring or perming (see also *Colouring – A Salon Handbook* and *Perming and Straightening – A Salon Handbook*). The woven strands should be cut considerably shorter than the overall length of the hair if a substantial amount of texturising and lift is required. The width between the weaving should be evenly spaced. To achieve heavy texturising, weave

Fig. 5.13 Weave cutting, using the closed scissors to weave out hair. The result is on the right; shorter hairs are dispersed amongst the longer ones.

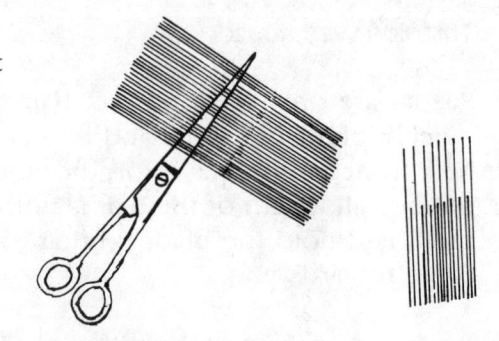

out the woven strands thickly. For a more subtle effect, weave the strands so that they are fine. Weave cutting can be carried out over the whole head, but it is very time-consuming because such narrow meshes (about 1cm) are used. Therefore weave cutting is usually restricted to specific areas.

(2) Chipping

This technique reduces bulk and weight from the points creating uneven hair lengths at the ends of the hair. The hair is held taut in vertical meshes and the points of the blades are pushed into the hair to cut out notches, as shown in Fig. 5.14.

Fig. 5.14 Chipping the hair with the points of the scissor blades creates uneven hair lengths at the ends of the hair.

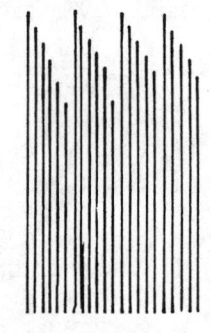

(3) Channel cutting

This technique involves taking a mesh and cutting it short, followed by taking the next mesh and leaving it long. This continues throughout the style, short followed by long, short followed by long, etc. This creates wide, visible channels of shorter hair through a style, which works particularly well on Afro hair for unusual effects.

(4) Pointing

The pointing technique of cutting uses only the points of the scissors. The scissors are lightly skimmed over the hair to soften the hard lines and to create wispy effects while removing as much bulk as necessary. Placing the index finger on the pivot of the scissors helps maintain control and balance of your movements when doing this on fringes. See Fig. 5.15 for how to hold sections vertically and point: this can be done all over the head, removing as much bulk as required.

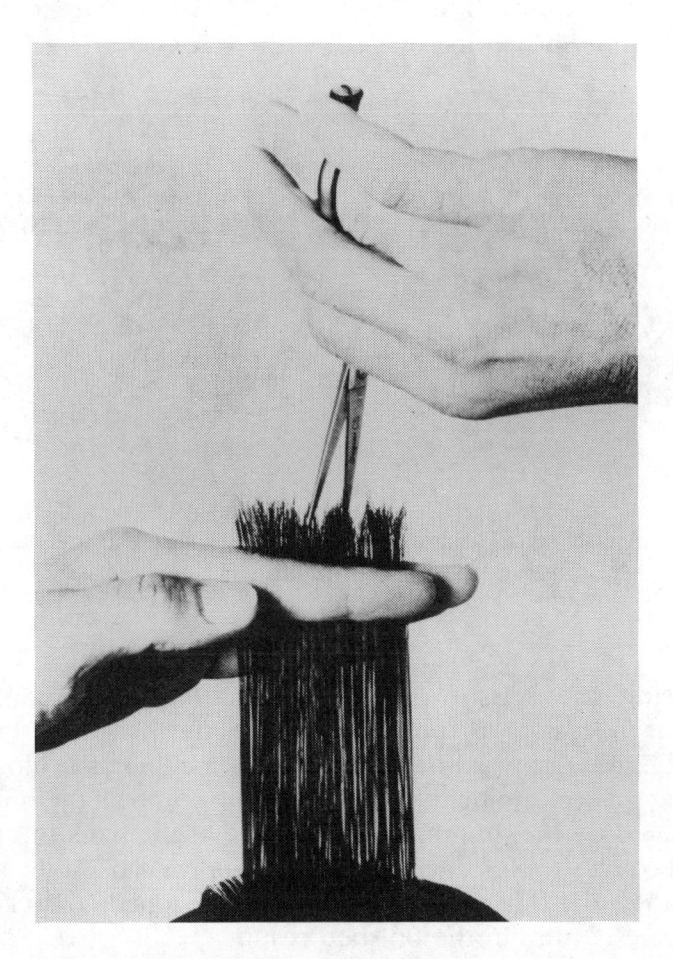

Fig. 5.15 Vertical point cutting technique using conventional scissors. (Courtesy of Rand Rocket Ltd.)

5.6 The scissor over comb technique (shingling)

A shingle or semi-shingle haircut describes a style which is graduated close into the nape of the neck following the contours of the head. The difference between the two cuts is that a shingle is graduated higher up the head than a semi-shingle. These styles were at the height of their popularity between the First and Second World Wars. Today, the term 'scissors over comb' describes this close graduating cutting technique and is used extensively in both men's and ladies' hair shaping to create short, close cut areas, as shown in Fig. 5.16.

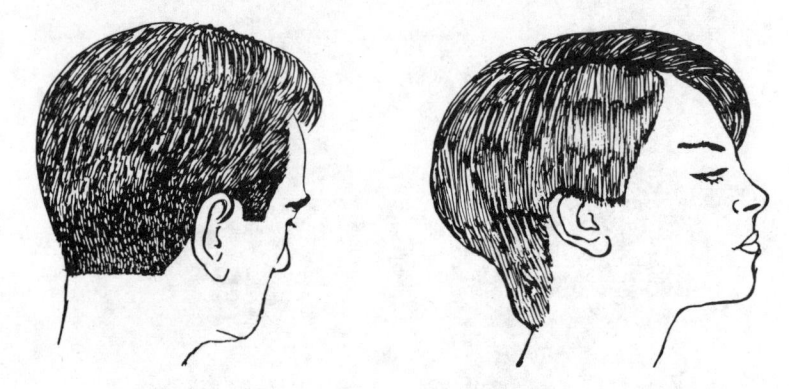

Fig. 5.16 A lady's and a man's style, created using the scissor over comb technique (also called shingling).

When using the scissor over comb cutting technique, a flowing movement is necessary to prevent steps in the hair. The thin, flexible comb is used in an upward direction, lifting the hair as it moves through the hair. The scissors are held parallel with the comb all the time. Only the blade, operated by the thumb, should move. As the hairs slip through the teeth of the comb they are cut off. Electric clippers can also be used for this as shown in Fig. 5.17. In this example, a wide-toothed comb is being used to create more texture in the finished result.

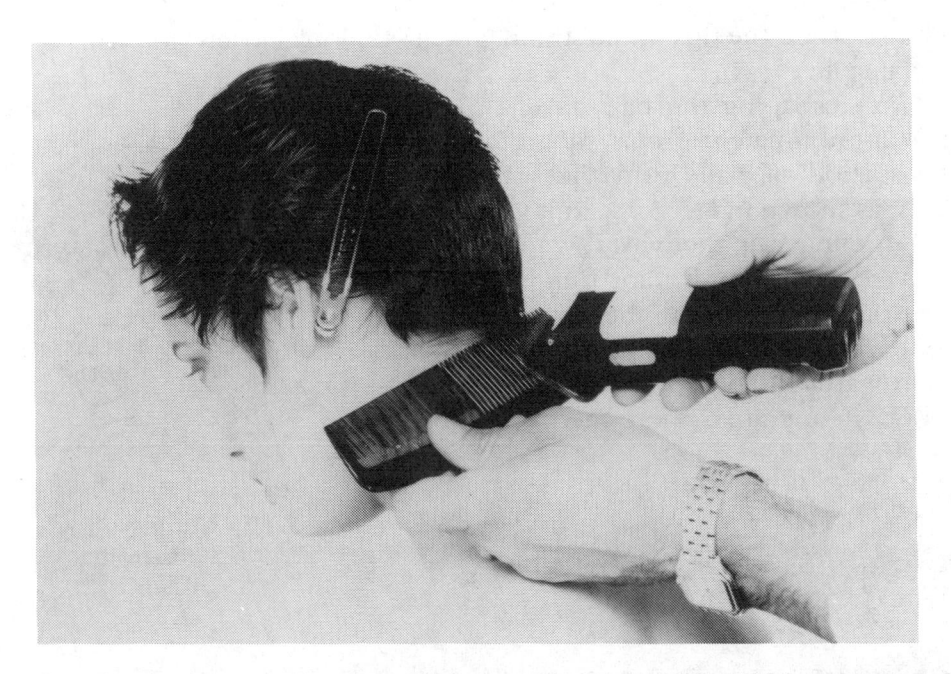

Fig. 5.17 Clipper-over-comb technique to give strong effect on nape. (Courtesy of Rand Rocket Ltd.)

5.7 Cutting split ends

Split ends or *Fragilitis crinium*, can be permanently cured in one way only – by cutting them off! If they are not cut off, the split will continue along the whole hair shaft. A split end is shown in Fig. 5.18. Long hair usually suffers from split ends because the ends are older and drier with a greater tendency to become brittle, and therefore split. We, as hairdressers, can easily remove split ends with scissors, but how much better it would be if we educated our clients in home hair-care to prevent them occurring so readily. See Chapter 7 on treatments.

Fig. 5.18 A split end.

Removing split ends from long hair is not usually just a matter of giving the hair a good one length cut. As split ends occur where tight elastic bands have been used, or areas where the hair is generally abused, split ends can usually be seen on the shorter hair strands as well. They will look like white dots on the tips of the strand, and if you look closely you will see the actual split.

After reshaping the hair, take a mesh of hair approximately 3 cms square and twist the section of hair from the scalp to the ends, as shown in Fig. 5.19. Run your thumb and forefinger up the twist towards the scalp to make the hair ends stand out. Beginning at the root end, cut off the protruding split ends with the points of your scissors, working towards the hair points. Repeat this procedure in any area where the hair is split.

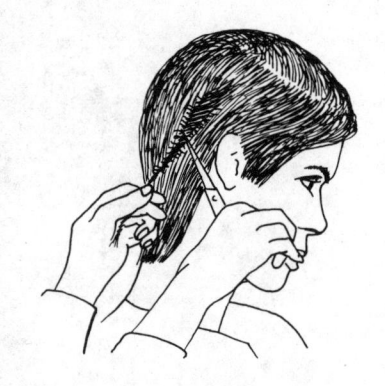

Fig. 5.19 Cutting off split ends from a twist of hair.

5.8 Cutting super curly hair

The term 'super curly' is used to describe hair which has a high degree of curl. It is usually seen on black people and is therefore often referred to as Afro or black hair (not the colour!). Many white people have super curly hair as well. Most people with such hair are reluctant to have it cut because it generally has a slower apparent rate of growth than straighter hair. Super curly hair still requires regular cutting, however, to keep it looking well-groomed and to maintain its condition and strength. Because this type of hair does not retain moisture very well, it is particularly prone to damage if it has been chemically relaxed, permed or frequently pressed with hot irons.

What do we mean by Afro hair?

Once super curly hair has been chemically relaxed or permed it is no longer described as being Afro. Afro hair is natural hair which is usually cut into a particular shape and allowed to dry naturally, so it requires different cutting techniques.

How is Afro hair prepared for cutting?

Afro hair is always cut when it is dry, preferably after shampooing and natural drying. Use a wide-toothed comb or pick to lift the hair out from the head and to remove any tangles in the hair. The comb is inserted into the hair and pulled out in an upwards movement with a turn of the wrist. When the hair is completely disentangled and standing away from the head it is ready for cutting. Spraying the hair lightly with an instant moisturising spray will make it easier to comb because this product coats each strand of hair with a lubricating film of oil.

What tools are used for cutting Afro hair?

Afro hair cannot be combed using a conventional cutting comb because it would pull and stretch the hair beyond its natural elastic limit, causing hair breakage. Therefore a wide-toothed Afro comb or pick is used along with conventional scissors or electric clippers (or both).

Afro hair cutting techniques

The complete haircut can be carried out using a free-hand cutting technique or the hair can be cut by lifting the hair with the comb and then cutting over the comb.

(a) Free-hand cutting technique using scissors
The hair is shaped beginning either at the nape or the front hairline. The stylist should constantly check the emerging hair shape and balance of the style by continually lifting the hair with the comb or pick. Standing back from the client will help the stylist see the overall shape and balance more easily.

(b) Free-hand cutting techniques using clippers
The hair is lifted out with a comb or pick before cutting. The cut can begin either at the nape or the front hairline. The clippers are carefully run over the hair making sure that an even shape and balance is maintained. During cutting, the stylist should continually lift the hair.

(c) Scissor/clipper over the comb technique
Starting at either the nape or front hairline, insert the comb or pick into the hair with the teeth down. Gently lift the hair out from the head and cut the hair that is extending beyond the teeth of the comb with either scissors or clippers.

Technical tips on cutting Afro hair

- Spraying with an instant moisturiser will make the hair easier to comb.
- Use clippers to shape hairlines (see [5.9]).
- Allow for greater spring in black hair than other hair.

- Avoid the use of razors as they tend to slice the hair making it more difficult to keep the hair in good condition.
- When cutting an Afro, continually lift out the hair and check the shape and balance of the style.
- It is easier to cut an Afro using scissors with long blades as less cuts have to be made.

5.9 Introduction to hairline shaping

Nowadays, hair is usually cut while it is wet after shampooing. Most texturising and thinning techniques are carried out when the hair has naturally dried out during the haircut, being easily re-dampened by a water spray for blow drying, setting or perming.

Although a prior examination of the hair and scalp and discussion between stylist and client should precede any hairdressing service, it is much easier to see the true lie of the hair (i.e. hair growth patterns) when the hair is wet. This is because styling methods often distort the natural lie of the hair and force it into opposite directions. For example, a client may part her hair on the side she has worn the parting since childhood, but it may be the opposite side to where the parting falls naturally.

Generally speaking, a style should work with the growth patterns of the hair so that it falls and moves in the direction that it grows naturally. By working to this formula, the style will be manageable and lasting. A cowlick on the front hairline can be a problem if the stylist tries to conceal it. As it is a strong growth of hair growing in an opposite, or unusual direction, it is not easily hidden. It is better practice to make the cowlick a feature of the haircut, by using the strong growth patterns for movement and direction.

The direction of hair cannot be altered by anything the hairdresser can do, as it is determined by the hair follicle, where our skills and products cannot reach. Therefore, cutting the hair to the same level as the skin surface will not make it grow back in a different direction, or indeed grow any thicker, faster or darker. Occasionally, it may be necessary to create a false hairline for a client whose hairline is either the wrong shape, or grows too weakly for the intended look. It may be that there are just a few hairs which grow too low for the style at the nape. This is very often carried out on black hair designs to create a strong, geometric shape on hairlines which are weak at the sides, nape and front.

Three different tools can be used when hairline shaping:

(a) clippers;
(b) razor;
(c) scissors.

Cutting 121

Great care should be taken to observe any pimples or other raised areas of skin which could be caught by the cutting tool. Always use a neck brush to brush away all hair clippings continually.

(a) Hairline shaping using clippers

There are many different types of hair clippers, but for this type of work an extremely fine blade is necessary so that it cuts close to the skin. Some clippers have adjustable blades while others may have interchangeable blades. The size of blade recommended for hairline shaping is 0000, which is equivalent to 0.1 mm. The clippers are directed against the natural lie of the hair towards the outline shape of the style as shown in Fig. 5.20. A line can be made with the very edge of the clippers to mark out the new shape before cutting. When shaping the front hairline with clippers, cover the client's eyes with tissue to prevent small hair clippings from entering the eyes.

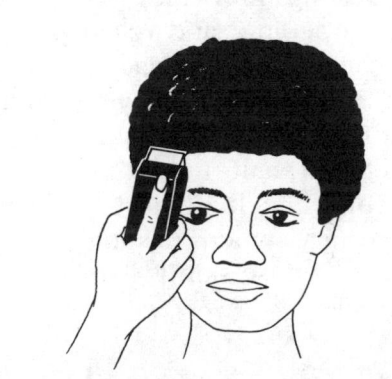

Fig. 5.20 Hairline shaping using electric hair clippers.

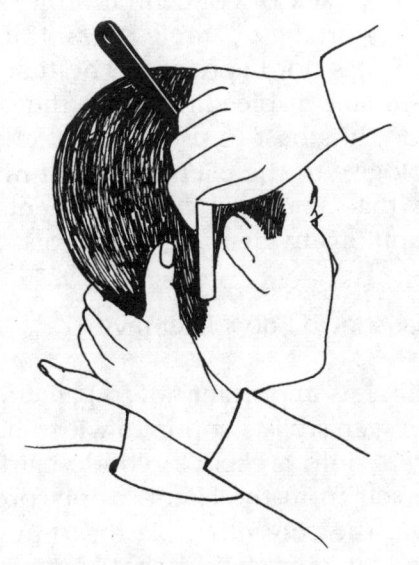

(b) Hairline shaping using a razor

The skin must be made wet and lubricated with a shaving cream or foam to help the razor glide close to the skin and facilitate the cutting of the hair. Any pimples or raised areas should be marked by removing the cream or foam so that they are left exposed (never rely on memory!). The razor is rested against the skin and brought down in a stroking movement while keeping the head still and the skin taut, as shown in Fig. 5.21. This takes considerable care and skill.

Fig. 5.21 Hairline shaping using a razor.

(c) Hairline shaping using scissors

It usually takes longer to carry out hairline shaping using scissors than it does with clippers, but women do not usually like the idea of having their hairline clippered or shaved. This probably comes from the myth that hair cut in this way grows back coarser or darker. The outline shape of the hairline is first cut with the scissors as shown in Fig. 5.22 and then the unwanted hair below this line is cut away by resting the blades flat on the skin and opening and closing quickly; moving only the blade operated by the thumb. When carrying out this fast cutting action, the skin should be stretched taut to avoid cutting the client's neck. This is especially necessary when dealing with older clients whose skin is looser and more wrinkled.

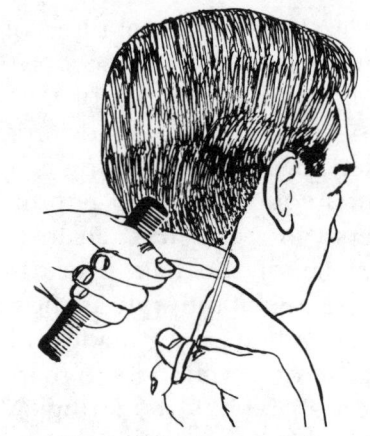

Fig. 5.22 Hairline shaping using scissors.

What should I do if I accidentally cut the client?

Accidents with scissors, razors or clippers can and do happen. It can be due to a lack of concentration for a split second, the stylist being jogged while working or carelessness. If it does happen, do not panic or pretend that it has not happened. The first thing to do is to apply pressure to the cut to stop it bleeding. With the possibility of infection being spread by blood, it is best to use a pad of damp cotton wool to apply the pressure. Apologise to the client, without making a major drama of the event! The fact that you can cut the client should help reinforce the need for scrupulous hygiene of your tools.

What should I do if I cut myself?

Again, it is important not to panic or pretend that it has not happened. We have seen stylists continue with a haircut with blood streaming down their fingers onto a client's blonde hair! Stop what you are doing and excuse yourself from the client. Apply pressure to the cut until clotting occurs. Cover the cut with a plaster to prevent hair clippings, products or client blood (if you should slip!) entering the cut. If a cut is severe medical treatment may be necessary. A plastic finger cot can be worn over a more severe cut that needs bandaging, although this may restrict your manipulative skills somewhat.

5.10 Technical haircutting tips

- During a haircut, stand away from your client occasionally as it is easier to identify any discord or disproportion from a distance.
- Use a vent brush to brush hair in different directions during a haircut so that you can see how well the hair is falling and any imperfections can be seen and corrected.
- Keep a water spray close at hand to redampen the hair during cutting if necessary.
- Work with the growth of the hair – not against it.
- Use the mirrors around the salon to check the shape of your haircut from different angles and distances.
- To check the base line of a short bob, a hand-mirror can be placed under the hairline to reflect any imperfections.
- When checking an Afro haircut stand at your client's side and slowly tilt the head away from you and then back again, keeping your eye on the outline shape.
- Keep your sections narrow so that the cutting line of the previous mesh can clearly be seen.
- Do not use tension on the hair when cutting over the ear. Make allowances for the degree of ear protrusion by allowing the hair to fall naturally and cutting free-hand in this area.
- Incorporate different cutting techniques in a style to achieve interesting and personalised hair designs.
- Remember that hair stretches more when it is wet so it will appear shorter when it has dried.

5.11 Trevor Sorbie — step by step

This series of step by step photographs shows how Trevor creates texture in a short head of hair, achieving interesting movement and varying hair length for a short tousled look.

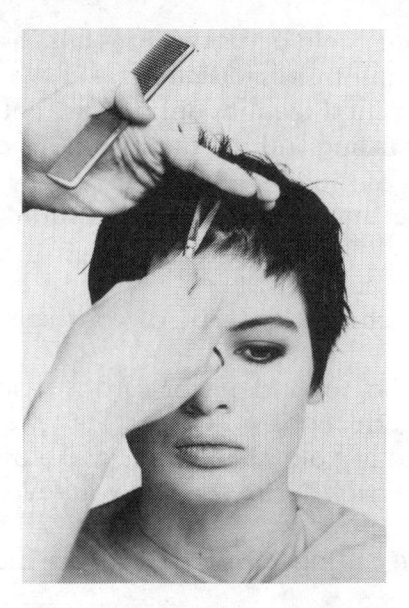

Step 1. Ordinary cutting scissors are used for this haircut to reduce the length and to create the texture. Starting at the front, the hair is cut to about 4 cms long. Using the points of the scissors the hair is chopped to achieve a variation in length and less weight at the ends of the hair.
(Photographs courtesy of Trevor Sorbie.)

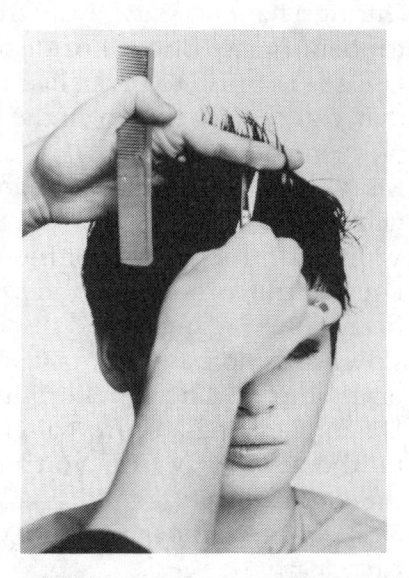

Step 2. Working towards the crown, the sections are taken the same as in step 1, reducing the bulk on the ends and creating texture by chopping into the hair.

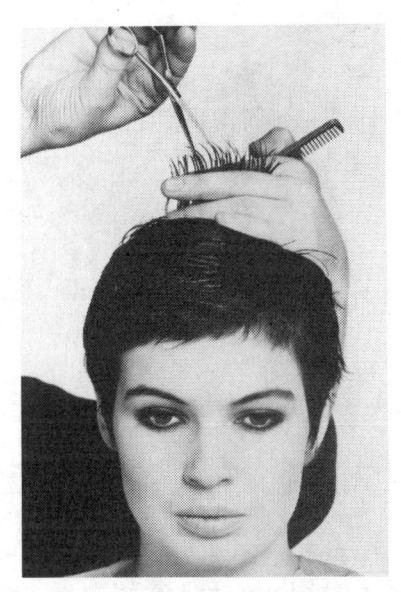

Step 3. Arriving at the crown, the overall length should be approximately 4–5 cms.

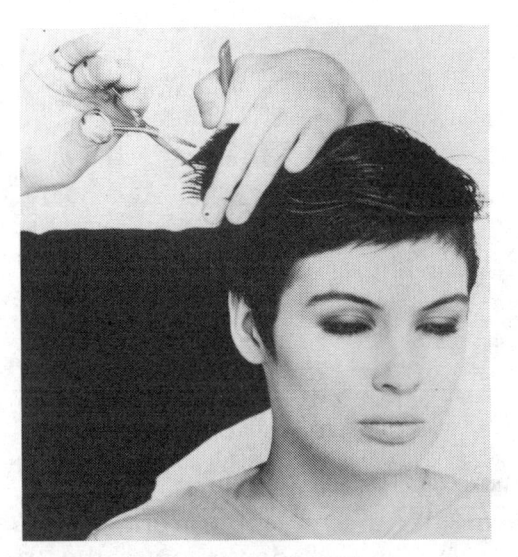

Step 4. The sides should be cut to approximately 2–3 cms long. Again, the points of the scissors are used to cut into the ends of the hair to create texture.

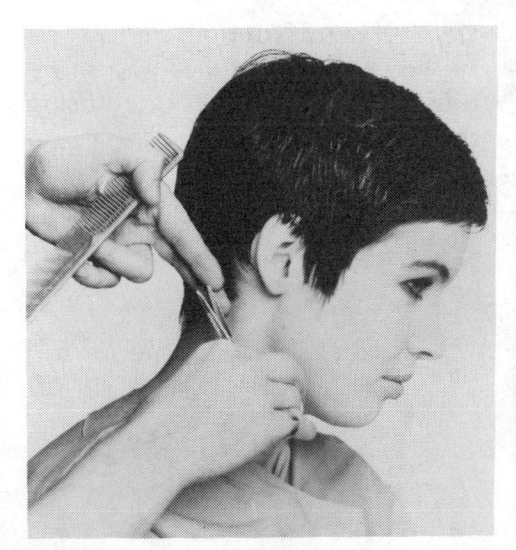

Step 5. Now working into the back area, the hair is cut short into the nape.

Step 6. The hair at the hairline is cut into a solid V shape.

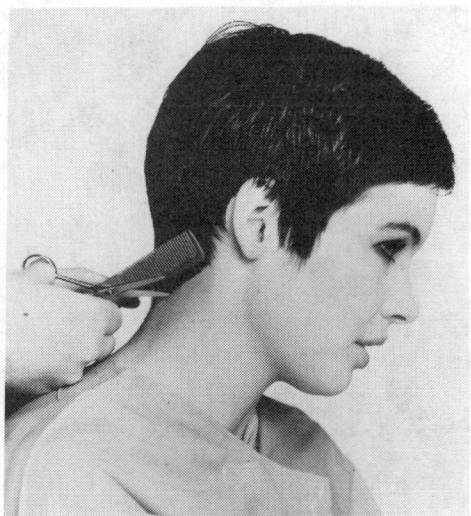

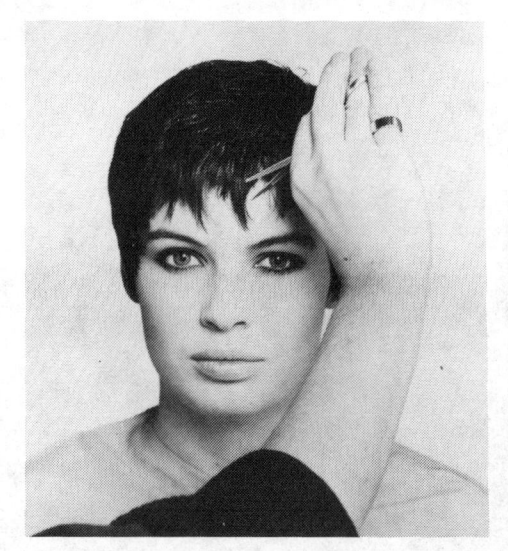

Step 7. Returning to the front, the hair is combed down onto the forehead. Using the freehand cutting technique (i.e. not holding the hair in the fingers) the hair is cut to leave a random cut look.

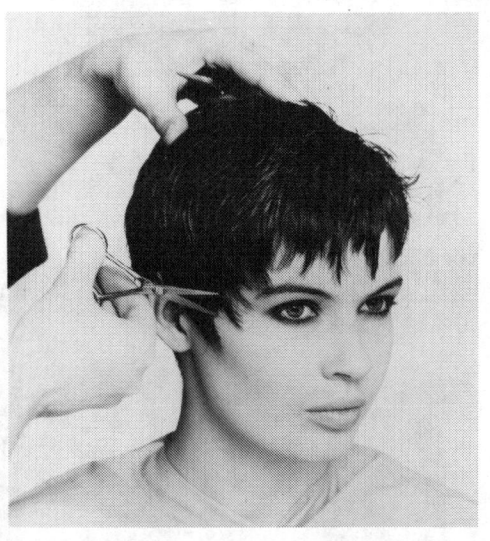

Step 8. The sides are cut using the same technique as used for the fringe.

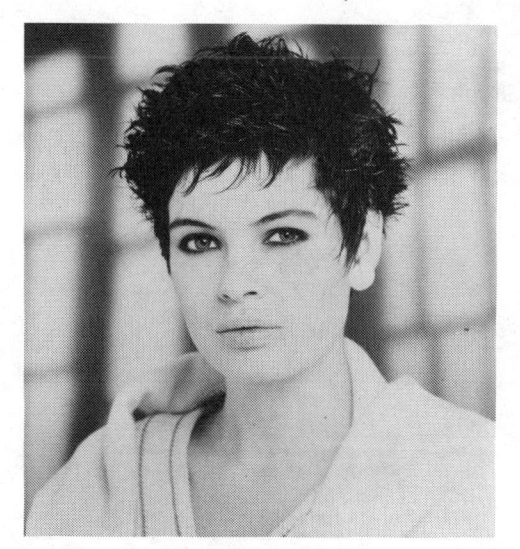

Step 9. Extra strength mousse is applied to give a fuller and more tousled effect and it is dried using the fingers.

Cutting 127

5.12 Alan International — step by step

The hair in the following photographs was cut by Jo Jordan, member of the artistic team of the Alan International hairdressing schools and academy, London. They show how a mid-length growing-out bob can be transformed into a strong design which has a contrast of length.

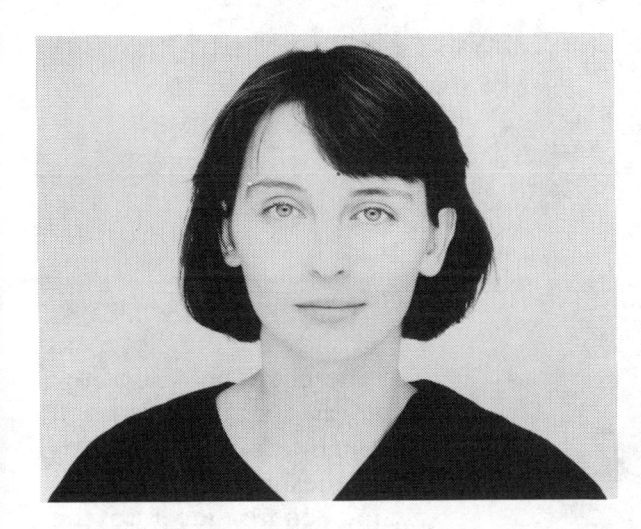

Step 1. Fine textured hair worn in a fringed, growing-out bob. The new look will have a short, flat fringe that curves around the forehead. Long pieces will be left in the cheek area for softness and the hair will be cut so that the under-sections will kick out to provide width. Before cutting, the hair was partially permed using the Sellotape technique (see *Perming and Straightening – A Salon Handbook*) which provides the root lift and movement necessary on the sections underneath.
(Photographs courtesy of Alan International.)

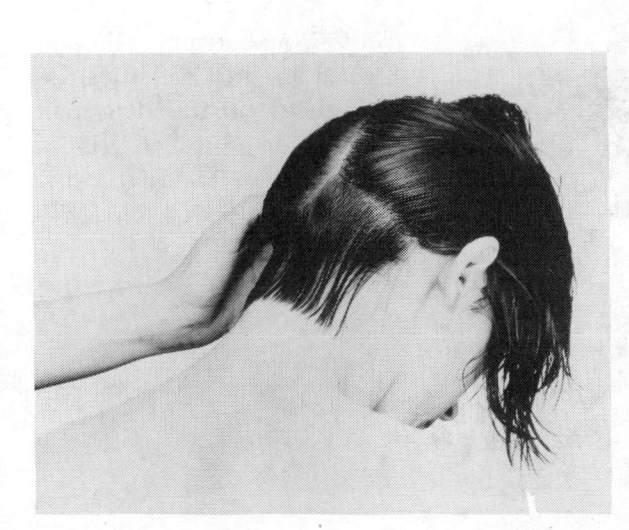

Step 2. The back of the hair is divided by a centre parting that runs from the crown to the nape. A semi-circular section is made running across the top of the occipital bone from one side to the other.

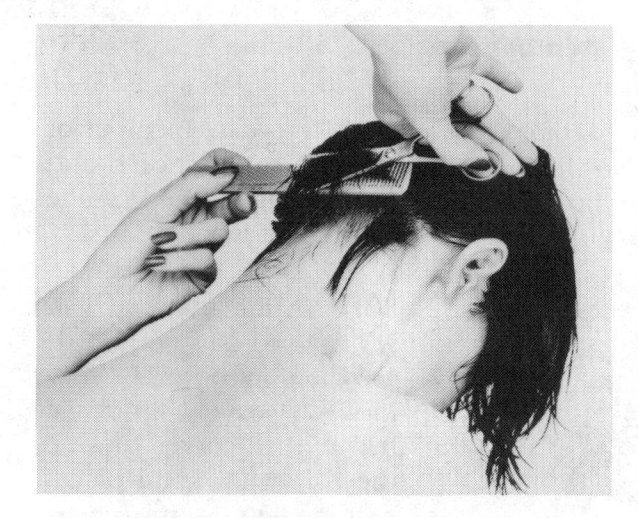

Step 3. The hair is cut in this section using the scissor over comb technique. Jo used thinning scissors for this to give a softer texture to the hair.

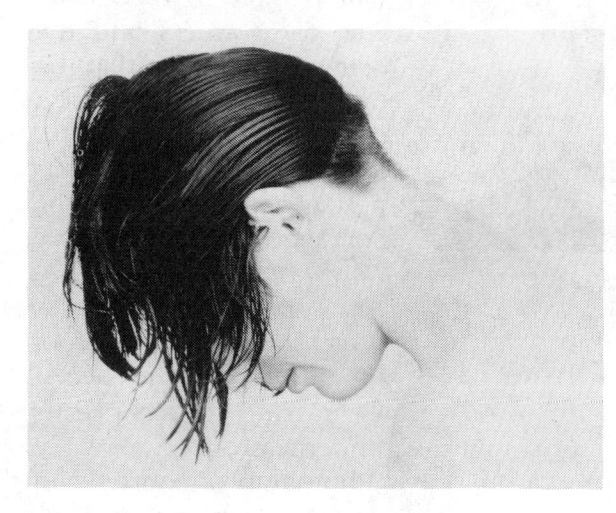

Step 4. The completed section showing the closeness of the cut. The rest of the hair at the back is then brought down using narrow meshes and cut to the same length, level to the top of the short underneath hair. This technique develops and builds a heavyweight line.

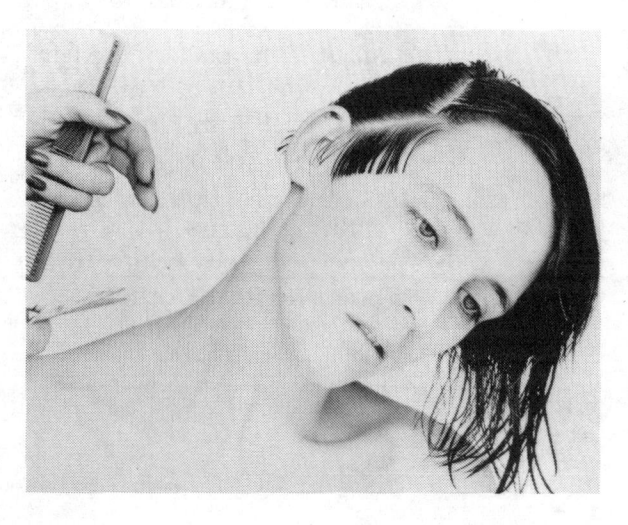

Step 5. A section is taken at the sides and the mesh is cut short on the diagonal. The over-lying lengths of hair are left longer for softness.

Cutting 129

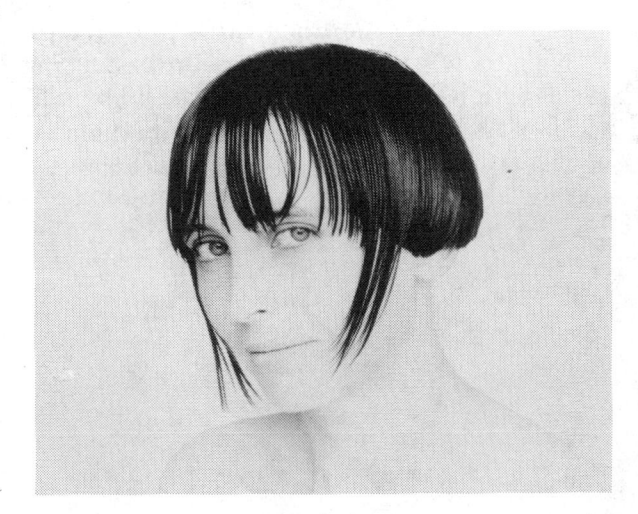

Step 6. Only the fringe to cut now. This photograph shows the longer lengths of hair left at the sides covering the shorter lengths underneath.

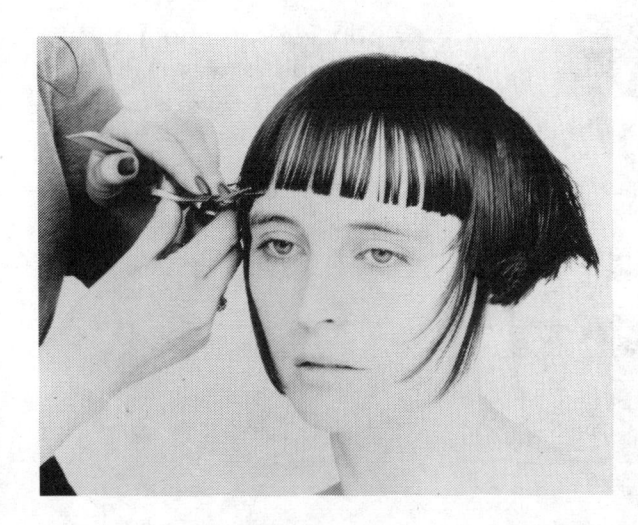

Step 7. The fringe is cut on a curve across the forehead using the free-hand cutting technique to achieve precision.

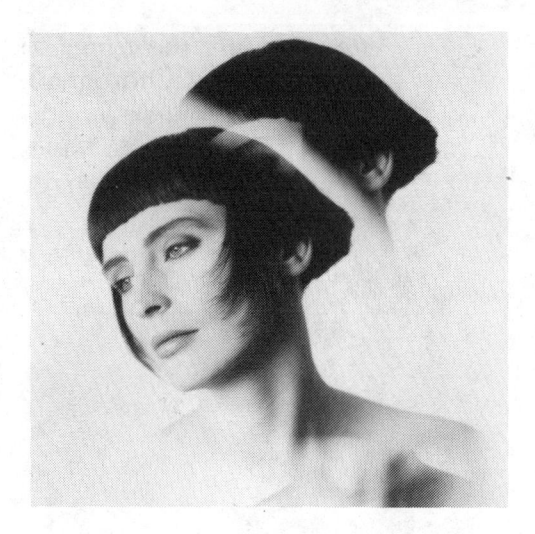

Step 8. In this photograph the hair was dressed using an oily wax which was smoothed over the hair for a sleek effect.

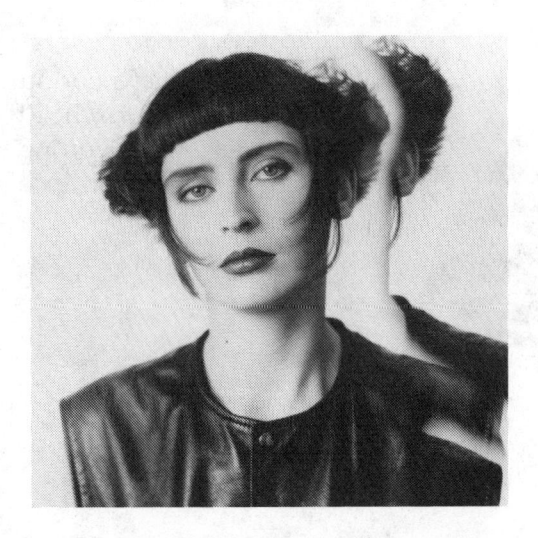

Step 9. For a dressier effect, pomade was applied to the hair and it was then blow dried up, away from the head.

5.13 Children's haircutting

The technique and procedures for cutting children's hair are basically the same as those for adults and adolescents. There are some differences, however, so stylists should be aware of the following:

(a) children's hair texture;
(b) hair-care for children;

(c) cutting techniques related to child behaviour;
(d) style lines for girls, boys and toddlers.

(a) Hair texture

Babies are born with soft, downy hair which will only last between one and four years before it is replaced with slightly coarser hair. The first 'baby hair' is often a different colour to the hair that replaces it and may also be more curly. The stylist should therefore inform the parent of the child that the curls may not return once cut.

(b) Hair-care

If the hair is to be cut whilst wet, use a low pH shampoo, and if possible, one which will not sting the eyes if it should accidentally come into contact with them (baby shampoo). Conditioner is not normally necessary because their hair will not have been abused at a young age.

Never carry out any form of chemical treatment on a child such as perming, tinting, bleaching or relaxing. The risks are too great for any stylist.

Cut the hair so that it will dry naturally and fall easily into place; parents do not want to have to style the hair with blow driers or tongs each time it is washed. Always check for the presence of nits, as it is very common amongst young children (see *Hygiene – A Salon Handbook*).

(c) Child behaviour

The first haircut a child has can be an extremely traumatic experience if enough patience, consideration and care are not taken. The child should visit the salon with the mother beforehand so that the salon becomes a familiar environment and the staff are not strangers. The child will be fascinated by what is going on, will see mother having her hair cut, shampooed etc., and see that she enjoys it.

When the child eventually visits the salon for the first haircut, the stylist must be friendly. Call the child by his or her first name or nickname as it will help the child to relax. A little bribery in the form of a small present or sweets works wonders!

Once the child is in the chair, make sure they are comfortable and that there is something to amuse them. Some salons have specially fitted out areas with chairs made to look like animals and have cartoons running on a video, with bright pictures on the walls.

Leave the child's hands free from underneath the gown so that they feel less confined and can amuse themselves with, perhaps, a small toy. Always treat the hair gently; any pulling will upset the child. If you plan to wet the hair using a spray gun, show the child how it works before using it. The same applies to the action of the scissors because it is often the noise of the scissor blades when they close that frightens children.

The biggest problem that a stylist faces is the child's inability to sit still. Try to carry out the haircut as quickly as possible and use your hand to steady the head by gently holding the chin or nape of the neck. Try to keep hair clippings from falling on the face and always balance your scissors and practise caution when shaping fringes and around the ears. Children have a natural tendency to make sudden, unexpected movements! Avoid any sudden movements yourself which might frighten the child.

(d) Style lines

Simple styles that follow the natural hair growth pattern are best for children because the hair will retain its shape throughout the day. Fringes are particularly popular for young children.

Blunt (club) cutting is recommended for children's hair because it helps make the hair look thicker and gives the ends more body. Razor cutting children's hair is not recommended as usually they do not like the slight dragging sensation caused by the razor. Thinning scissors or texturising techniques can be used on children's hair if it is particularly dense.

If the hair is long, spend a long time showing the mother how different styles can be achieved, such as ponytails, plaits, bunches, etc. Also show how to use and place slides and ribbons. A warning about traction alopecia would not be amiss (refer to *Hygiene – A Salon Handbook*).

5.14 Questions

1. Why is it impossible to do the same cut on every head?
2. Why should you not only learn cutting techniques which are in fashion?
3. What are the differences between the three main cutting methods?
4. What is 'club' cutting and when would you use it?
5. What is 'taper' cutting and when would you use it?
6. Giving reasons, which type of cutting would you use before a perm?
7. How does backcombing affect a taper cut?
8. Why do you razor cut wet hair?

Cutting 133

9 What two ways can you use a razor to taper cut?
10 How do you club cut with a razor?
11 What is 'thinning' the hair?
12 Do single or double notch blades remove more hair?
13 How are thinning scissors different to conventional scissors?
14 Where should you avoid using thinning scissors?
15 How would you thin hair all over a head?
16 How would you thin hair with conventional scissors?
17 How would you thin hair with a razor?
18 What is weave cutting?
19 What is chipping?
20 When might you use channel cutting?
21 What is pointing?
22 Where would you use scissor over comb cutting?
23 How do you prevent steps in the hairline?
24 Describe how you would cut split ends off a client's hair.
25 What is super curly hair?
26 What is Afro hair?
27 How should Afro hair be prepared for cutting?
28 What tools are used for cutting Afro hair?
29 Why can't a conventional cutting comb be used?
30 Describe the techniques for cutting Afro hair using scissors and clippers.
31 Briefly list the main technical tips when cutting black hair.
32 What do we mean by hairline shaping?
33 Why can we not permanently alter the direction of hair growth?
34 Describe hairline shaping using clippers, razors and scissors. What precautions would you take when using these instruments (if any)?
35 What action should be taken if you cut a client?
36 What would you do if you cut yourself?
37 List what you consider as the most important six haircutting tips.
38 Why should you warn a mother before cutting a child's curls?
39 Why should a special shampoo be used on a child?
40 How can you introduce children to a salon?
41 Why does the behaviour of a child matter when cutting their hair?
42 List some of the things you would remember to do when cutting a child's hair.
43 Why should the style lines for a child follow the natural lines of the hair?
44 What type of cutting method is particularly suitable for a child's hair?
45 Why should you check children for head lice before starting a service?

6 Setting and Blow Drying

Both setting and blow drying involve a temporary change in the structure of the hair. Wet hair is stretched around rollers or with a brush and dried in its stretched state. The degree of curl introduced into the hair is always slightly tighter than actually desired, so that the hair can be brushed out into the planned style. The hair remains in this stretched position until it is wet again. Because no chemical reaction has taken place the change is physical; it involves only a change in the shape of the keratin, and can easily be reversed. This form of temporary set is known as a cohesive set. Because it is a physical change the hair can be set as frequently as desired. This is the basis of fingerwaving, pin curling, roller setting and all wet setting methods. The stylist should know whether each of these methods should be carried out individually on a head, or used in combination to produce the desired effect.

This chapter will examine what happens inside the hair and the various methods of setting and blow drying the hair that are available.

6.1 The cohesive set

As the setting of hair relies on its ability to stretch, setting can only be carried out really successfully on hair that is in good condition. The stretching of dry hair is controlled to a great extent by the weak, but numerous, hydrogen bonds which were described in [1.2], and illustrated in Fig. 1.3. Because there are millions of these bonds, they allow the hair to stretch slightly, while the stronger but less numerous disulphide bonds resist the movement. To obtain greater extension, the stretching is carried out on wet hair, by either winding tightly on rollers or by brushing when blow drying. Figure 6.1(a) shows dry hair in its unstretched state, with a hydrogen bond between the hydrogen and oxygen atoms. Figure 6.1(b) shows what happens when wet hair is stretched – water molecules enter the hydrogen bonds, allowing the hair to stretch further, and this is known as 'bound water'. During drying, the bound water is evaporated off. In Fig. 6.1(c) you can see that because the water is evaporated off while the hair is still in its stretched state, the bonds have reformed in different positions. When the rollers, or brush, are removed, the hair remains in its stretched state. It will not return to its normal state until the hair is wet, but because hair is hygroscopic (it absorbs moisture from the atmosphere – generally about 10 per cent of the cortex can be water) the cohesive set will be lost quickly unless it is protected from moisture. We therefore protect it with various setting agents such as setting and blow dry lotions, hairsprays, etc. If it were not protected the sequence shown in Fig. 6.1 would be reversed and the set would be lost.

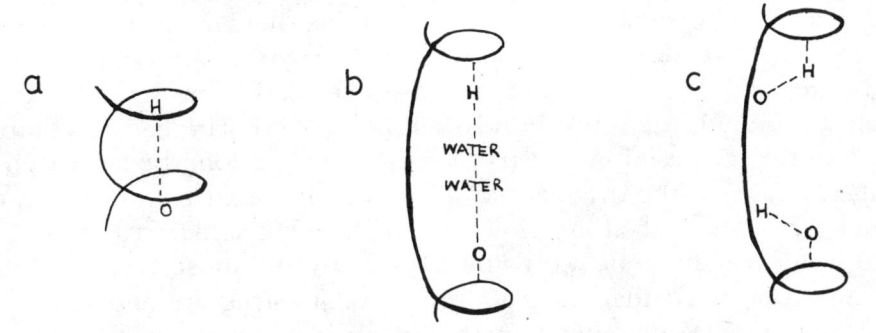

Fig. 6.1 (a) Hair in its unstretched state.
(b) Bound water enters the hair as it stretches.
(c) During drying water is evaporated off and the hair is held in its stretched state when bonds are formed in different positions.

What are the two types of keratin involved in a cohesive set?

You may have heard people talking about two types of keratin as if they were totally different things. These are the magical alpha- (α) and (β) beta-keratins. Put simply, alpha-keratin is keratin in its unstretched state, while beta-keratin is keratin in its stretched state. Alpha-keratin is rather like an unstretched spring, while beta-keratin is like a stretched spring. Remember that it is the spring-like structure of the cortex that gives hair its elasticity. Set hair is hair which has been dried in a stretched state, so it is beta-keratin. If it is wetted, it returns to being alpha-keratin. If you can remember from Fig. 1.3, there are still powerful disulphide bonds intact in the cortex which will help pull the hair back to its original shape once the new hydrogen bonds are broken by absorbed water. The two types of keratin are summarised below:

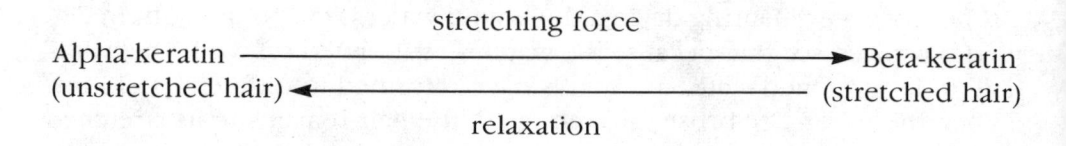

```
                          stretching force
Alpha-keratin        ─────────────────────────▶   Beta-keratin
(unstretched hair)   ◀─────────────────────────   (stretched hair)
                             relaxation
```

Is there a difference between the cohesive set and the heat setting carried out on dry hair with heated tongs?

The simple answer to this question is yes. The use of heated waving irons, tongs, crimpers, rollers etc. (see Chapter 3 for more detail) is often thought by hairdressers to work in exactly the same way. Hair is both heated and stretched at the same time and then held under tension until it is cool. The hydrogen bonds between the polypeptide chains of keratin are broken by both the heat and the tension placed on the hair. The greater the heat applied, the more bonds will be broken. The hair takes up the shape of the tool used. As the hair cools under tension, the hydrogen and oxygen atoms of the original bonds are too far apart to reform, so they form new bonds with atoms close by which keep the hair in its new shape. Cold water has little effect on a heat set; *hot* water must be used to break the new bonds so that the hair can relax its structure and reform the original bonds. Remember that too much heat setting will damage the cuticle of the hair.

What are the terms used to describe setting?

The French term for setting is *mise-en-pli*. This has led to the use of the shortened version 'pli', used to describe the placing of wet hair in position for drying. The following terms are used to describe the stages in the setting of hair:

First pli: wet hair in position (on rollers) ready for drying.
Second pli: dry hair after it has been dressed (the finished style).

> **A note on incorrect usage of the term 'pli'**
>
> Some stylists (and also teachers of hairdressing) use terms to describe the stages of setting which are *technically incorrect* as follows:
>
> *First pli*: wet hair in position ready for drying.
> *Second pli*: dry hair which is still in the setting position (still in rollers).
> *Third pli*: the final dressing.
>
> The term 'second pli' in the last example is also used in competition styling to mean deceiving the judges by carefully removing the hair from the rollers, pincurls, etc. partly dressing the hair and then replacing the rollers and clips back into the original set position. This saves time on the competition floor and also ensures that any faults in the pli are corrected in advance.

Only the terms first and second pli will be used in this book although they will often be replaced by the word 'set'.

6.2 Finger waving

Before rollers became popular in Britain during the fifties, all sets were achieved by using finger waves and pincurls. If you look at the movies of the thirties and forties you will be able to see the waves and curls created by these methods. The styles were relatively flat, compared with the degree of lift and volume that can be achieved by using rollers.

What is finger waving?

Finger waving is the art of shaping wet hair into waves using a comb and the fingers. Technically speaking, finger waving is the term used when the hair has been wetted and a setting aid (such as a lotion or gel) has been applied. (If a setting aid is not used, the process should be called water waving.) As the hair must be sufficiently wet and under control for finger waving, the application of a setting aid, such as a gel, is strongly recommended.

138 Cutting and Styling: a salon handbook

What effect does finger waving produce?

Finger waving produces S-shaped movements or waves in the hair. As the hair is moulded and shaped to the form of the head and the direction of the natural hair growth pattern, the finished look is close to the head with a minimum of volume. A drawing of a finger waved head is shown in Fig. 6.2. Finger waving is not successful on Afro hair unless a heavy dressing is used. This will stop the hair springing back because of its natural, tight curl formation.

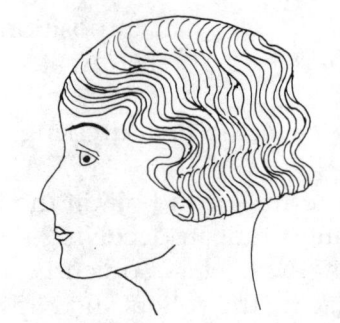

Fig. 6.2 A finger waved head.

A wave is made up of two raised *crests* and one dip between these, called a *trough*. These can be seen in Fig. 6.3. The distance between the crests should be approximately 30 mm and this is referred to as the *width of the wave* or *wave size*. The height of the crest and the depth of the wave is determined by the angle of combing. The *wave direction* is created by the angle at which the index finger is placed on the hair.

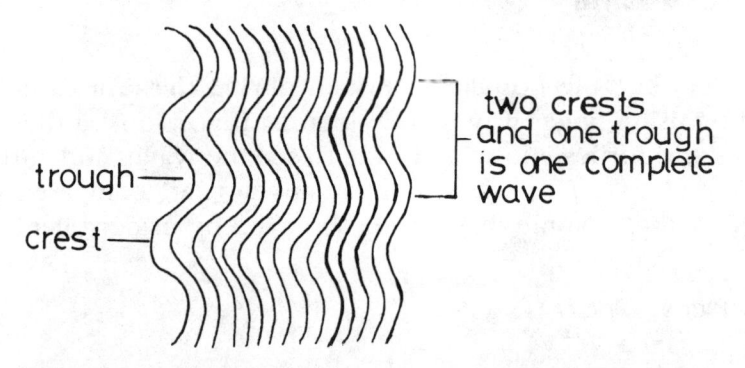

Fig. 6.3 Waves are made up of crests and troughs.

Why should a stylist learn finger waving?

Finger waving is an excellent introduction to setting hair because it is the skill of controlling and directing hair. It develops the discipline and manipulative skills necessary for hairdressing. Finger waving is often used in competition work, historical styles and displays. It is also seen occasionally in contemporary styling to create specific looks. Those wishing to enter the world of theatre, film and television as hair stylists need to be expert at finger waving, to have the ability to create styles of the past.

How is the hair prepared for finger waving?

After shampooing, disentangle the hair and apply a setting aid. Ensure that the hair is thoroughly wet and that the setting aid is evenly distributed on the hair. Using a straight comb, with both wide- and narrow-spaced teeth, mould the hair by combing into the intended direction. If waving with a parting, look for the hair growth direction to find where the hair parts naturally (see [4.6]) and distribute the hair out evenly from the parting. If you intend to wave without a parting to the side, comb the hair away from the face and direct the hair to the side of the head that you want the hair to go. For a style waved back from the face without any parting or sideways direction (this type of style being called a 'Pompadour'), comb the hair straight back from the face. Remember to keep the hair free from tangles and *wet*.

How should the comb be held for finger waving?

The comb should be held with the thumb and little finger on one side, with three fingers on the other. This is shown in Fig. 6.4. Holding the comb like this helps to make the waving easier, because you will have full control over the comb.

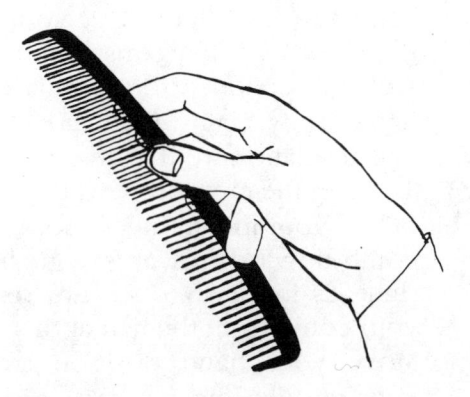

Fig. 6.4 How to hold a comb for finger waving.

Guidelines for finger waving

- Keep your forearm up level with your hand when waving.
- Always stand immediately behind the portion of the head that you are waving.
- Hold the comb as shown in Fig. 6.4.
- Keep the hair wet during waving.

- Apply a setting aid to the hair.
- The hair should be cleanly combed away from the face before waving.
- If a parting is used, the hair should be evenly combed and distributed from the parting.
- Use only the index and second finger during waving.

Finger waving practice

Like many hairdressing skills, it is often better for the novice to practise on a tuition head, or hair weft, before progressing to a live model. As finger waving requires discipline, control and manipulative skills, it is suggested that the learner practises the following exercise before waving a full head.

Finger waving exercise on a tuition head or hair weft

(1) If using a hair weft, secure this to a malleable block using postiche pins. If using a tuition head, section off a section of hair at the back by making a parting across the back of the head from ear to ear, just below the crown area. Thoroughly comb the hair, wet it, and then apply a styling aid such as gel or setting lotion. The latter can easily be removed with warm water after the exercise.

(2) Comb the hair using a semicircular movement which will direct the hair over to the left. Place your index finger (of the hand not holding the comb) firmly against the head about 3 cms below the top of the weft or section, to keep this curve in position. While keeping the hand firmly against the head, draw your comb through the rest of the hair to make sure that the hair is still free from tangles.

(3) To form the crest of the wave, insert your comb approximately 2 cms below your index finger. Hold the comb flat to the head and push the comb upwards towards your finger, in a movement directed to the right, as in Fig. 6.5. Do not remove your comb from the hair at this stage. Move your hand position so that your middle finger is resting on the teeth of the comb. Your fingers will now hold the crest in position while you continue waving.

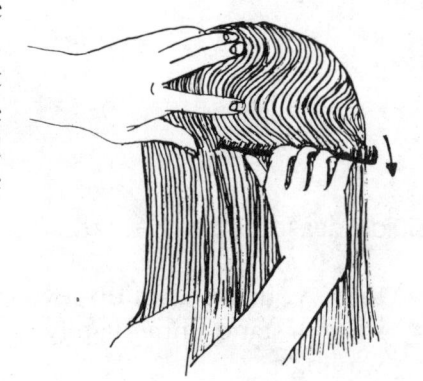

Fig. 6.5 Forming the crest of the wave using a comb.

(4) The second crest can now be formed by following exactly the same procedure, but directed to the left instead of to the right.
(5) These movements continue all the way down the hair until all the hair is waved.
(6) To finish the wave, use pincurls (see [6.3]) to curl the hair points up to the last wave crest, as shown in Fig. 6.6. Notice in the diagram that the pincurls are used to continue the wave movement by being directed clockwise because the last wave crest direction is to the left.

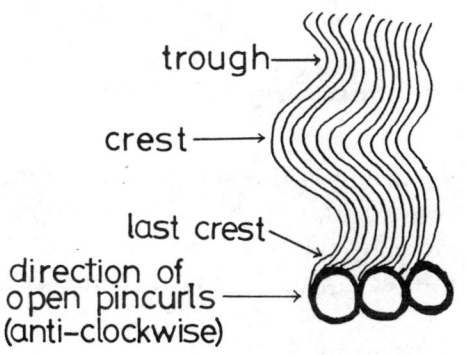

Fig. 6.6 Pincurling to the wave crest.

Finger waving a whole head

(1) Begin by finding the natural direction and fall of the hair as you would for finding a natural parting (see [4.6]). By doing this you will be able to see where the first wave should be placed, and you will have started the initial wave.
(2) Place your index finger below the crest you have just formed and your second finger above it. Increase the height of the crest by inserting your comb into the hair and pushing it upwards.
(3) Hold the crest in position, while you make the second movement in the opposite direction to the first.
(4) As your wave movements need to be continued around the head, you will need to join up the waves. This takes skill because a wave can be destroyed when attempting this if the comb and hair are not fully controlled. It is important that the waves moving in the same direction are joined so that the wave directions do not clash. It is more difficult to join up a narrow strip of waving to adjacent waves than it is to wave both sides of the head and join up down the back.
(5) When joining up in the crown area, the crest of the wave should be slightly faded to look more natural. This is called 'losing a wave' because the ridge is flattened so that it appears more natural.
(6) When the waving is complete, the hair at the sides and nape can be finished by pin curling to the last wave crest.
(7) Some stylists use clips to keep the hair in position for drying but these can cause marks on the hair. If the hair has to be secured, use tape

which can be gently pinned into position across the head in the troughs of the waves.

(8) After drying, comb the hair thoroughly, retracing the wave movements.

6.3 Pincurling

Pincurling is the sculpturing of wet hair into a series of wound coils to form a curl, which is secured in place by pins or clips before drying. There are many different types of pincurls that can be used to produce a variety of effects, but they do fall into two main categories:

(1) flat pincurls;
(2) stand-up pincurls.

(1) Flat pincurls

As the name implies, this type of pincurl is formed close to the head and is held in position using either pins or a clip, as shown in Fig. 6.7. There are four types of flat pincurls:

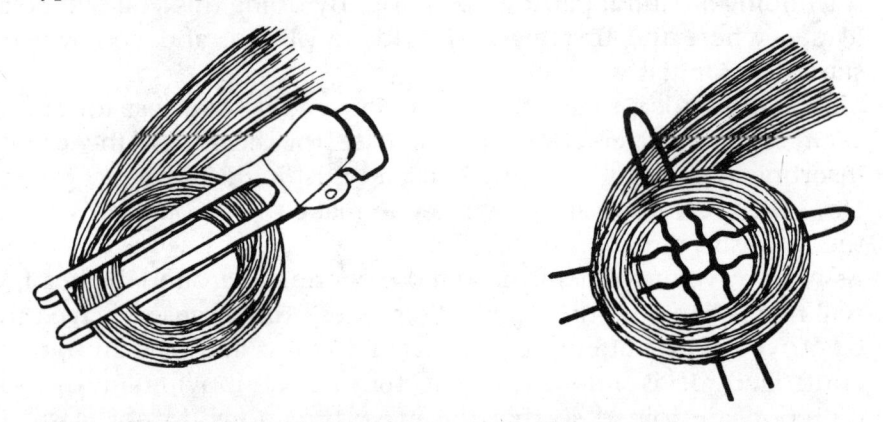

Fig. 6.7 Securing pincurls with either a clip or pins.

(a) open (barrelspring) pincurls;
(b) closed (clockspring) pincurls;
(c) reverse pincurls;
(d) long stem pincurls.

(a) Open (barrelspring) pincurls
Open pincurls (otherwise known as barrelspring curls because they resemble the shape of the spring used in hand hair clippers) have an open

centre, as shown in Fig. 6.8. They produce a soft, casual type of curl because it is formed so that each coil of hair is made the same size as the previous one. Therefore it produces an even wave formation throughout the hair's length, as can be seen again in Fig. 6.8. Open pincurls can be used to create soft movement when the hair is short because only one loop will be made. On longer hair, several loops will produce an effect similar to that of using rollers, but without the volume at the roots.

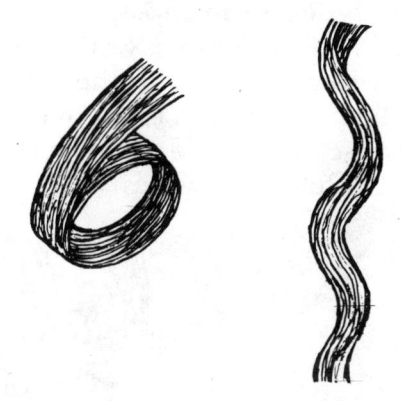

Fig. 6.8 The open or barrelspring pincurl, set on the left with the dressed result on the right.

(b) Closed (clockspring) pincurls
Closed pincurls (otherwise known as clockspring curls because they resemble the shape of a spring found in analogue watches) have a closed centre, as shown in Fig. 6.9. They produce a tight curl because it is formed so that each coil of hair is made smaller than the previous one, with the points of the hair ending in a small circle in the centre. Therefore, it produces a springy curl which gets tighter towards the ends, as can be seen again in Fig. 6.9. Closed pincurls are ideal for hair that drops easily, especially at the nape. However, this type of pincurl is often difficult to dress after drying if it has been used in areas where a flat open pincurl would have been better.

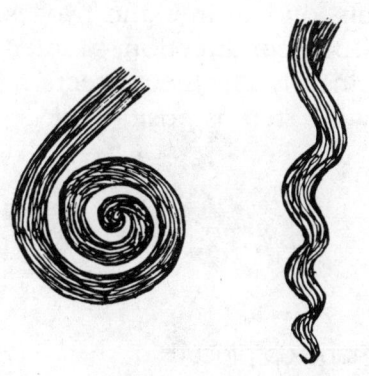

Fig. 6.9 The closed or clockspring pincurl, set on the left with the dressed result on the right.

(c) Reverse pincurls

Reverse pincurls are open, flat pincurls arranged in rows and directed clockwise and anticlockwise in each alternate row, as can be seen in Fig. 6.10. They produce a wave result similar to that of finger waving because each row is formed in the opposite direction to the last, as can be seen again in Fig. 6.10. Closed pincurls should not be used for reverse curling because they produce a curl formation which is too tight to dress successfully into waves.

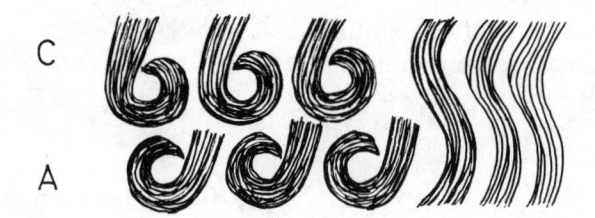

Fig. 6.10 Reverse pincurls and their result. C are clockwise pincurls while A are anti-clockwise pincurls.

(d) Long stem pincurls

Long stem pincurls have a long stem with less hair being looped to form the body of the curl, as shown in Fig. 6.11. The stem of the curl is usually gently curved rather than being left completely straight, to create loose wave movements, as can be seen again in Fig. 6.11. Long stem pincurls are particularly useful for creating flat curl results on hairlines and fringes.

N.B. Stem direction – remember that all pincurls take their direction from the way the stem is positioned.

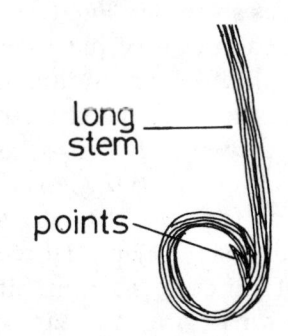

Fig. 6.11 A long stem pincurl.

(2) Stand-up pincurls

Stand-up pincurls produce volume at the roots because they sit on their own base in an upwards direction, so can be used instead of rollers to achieve lift. This is shown in Fig. 6.12. They can also be used as part of a pli that includes both rollers and pincurls. Sometimes the stand-up pincurls will require padding to maintain and support their shape. Cotton wool or crepe hair can be used for this purpose. As with all pincurls, it is important to make sure that the hair points are cleanly enclosed within the curl to avoid buckled ends. Also, clips and pins used to hold the pincurl in place must be carefully positioned so that the hair is not marked. For stand-up pincurls, the clip is slipped through the base of the curl so that it does not interfere with the body of the curl.

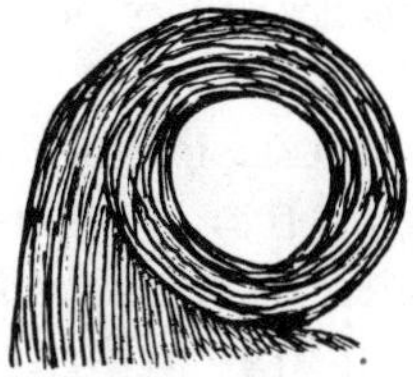

Fig. 6.12 The stand-up pincurl, which may require some padding.

It is possible to use pincurls for the whole set by incorporating different techniques to produce the desired volume, shape and curl. Alternatively pincurls and rollers may be used in unison as for a combination pli.

6.4 Roller setting

Roller setting is the term used to describe the wrapping of hair around cylindrical or conical-shaped rollers to produce varying degrees of volume, curl and wave.

Unfortunately, some stylists believe the misleading notion that setting hair on rollers requires the minimum of attention. This results in rollers being used in an uninteresting and unimaginative way, producing mundane shapes. Successful roller setting depends upon the stylist placing the rollers so that they produce the desired hair direction and movement. Time spent rolling up the hair will save time when the hair is dressed. If the hair is set in accordance with the direction of the finished style, the dressing will be easy. Conversely, if the hair is set in rollers without consideration to the finished look, the stylist will have to force the hair into the intended position, often disguising the faults with excess backcombing and hairspray. Obviously, the client will then find her hair difficult to manage because it will want to revert to the position in which it was set, rather than remaining in the forced direction it was placed in during the dressing. A thoughtful pli saves time later and is easier for the client to handle afterwards.

When should rollers not be used?

There are occasions when the desired effect can be more easily produced by using methods other than rollering. For example, if rollers are used at right angles to the hairline, unsightly breaks will appear in the final dressing, as shown in Fig. 6.13. The stylist will have to backcomb and tease the hair to correct this. How much easier it would be for the stylist (and the client) if pincurls had been used to create the intended direction and movement on the hairline.

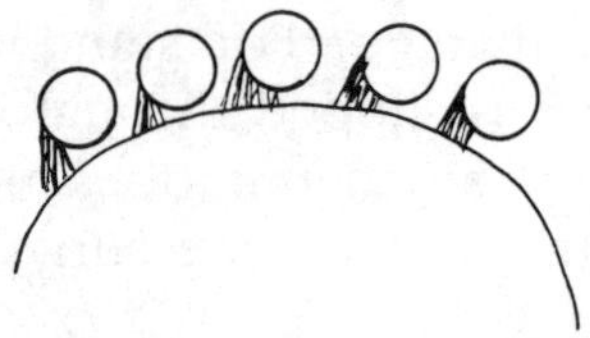

Fig. 6.13 Rollers placed at right angles to the hairline will produce breaks in the dressing.

What effects can be achieved using rollers?

The principles behind choosing the appropriate roller techniques depend on three main factors:

(1) how curly or straight the hair needs to be (roller size);
(2) the degree of volume required at the roots (volume control);
(3) the direction of the intended movement (roller direction).

(1) Choosing the appropriate roller size

The degree of curl or smoothness that is achieved is determined by the size of roller that is used. For example, a mesh of hair wrapped around a roller six times will produce a curlier effect than if it were wrapped around a larger roller twice. The larger the roller, the fewer times the hair can be wrapped around it, resulting in softer movement of hair. If the roller size is judged wrongly, the stylist will need to make corrections to the pli when dressing the hair. This could mean using tongs to strengthen the movement or stretching the hair straighter using a brush and blowdrier. Needless to say, practice makes perfect!

(2) Volume control

There are four variations of root volume that can be achieved using rollers. These are:

(a) normal volume (on-base);

(b) maximum volume (over-directed);
(c) minimum volume (under-directed);
(d) minimum volume on hairline (off-base).

To discuss each of these properly, we should first identify the vocabulary of roller setting terminology so that each of the above variations can be fully understood. 'Volume' means the amount of root lift (or bounce) that is achieved, producing varying degrees of width or height. A section of hair which is taken for a roller on which the roller will be positioned is called the 'base'. This section should be no wider than the length of the roller being used. The reason why should be obvious in Fig. 6.14!

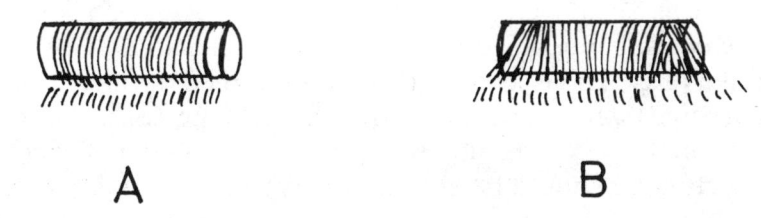

Fig. 6.14 (a) A correctly wound section.
(b) An incorrectly wound section because it is too wide.

(a) Normal volume is achieved by placing the roller so that it sits exactly on its own base, called an 'on-base roller'. The section must not be wider than the length of the roller being used and the base depth is equivalent to the roller's diameter (see Fig. 6.15). The roller can be used to measure the size of the base.

The on-base roller technique is probably the most common of all roller placements. It seems that many stylists do not place rollers in an imaginative way to create the varying degrees of volume required for a style.

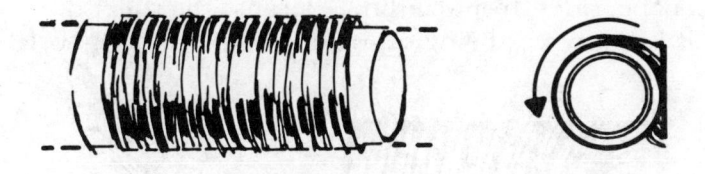

Fig. 6.15 On-base roller.

(b) Maximum volume is achieved by placing the roller so that it sits on the upper part of its base and is known as an over-directed roller. The base is equivalent to twice the diameter of the roller being used. Because the roller sits forward on the base maximum volume is achieved, and this is

shown in Fig. 6.16. This roller technique should be used when maximum lift is required, such as on the crown or front hairline.

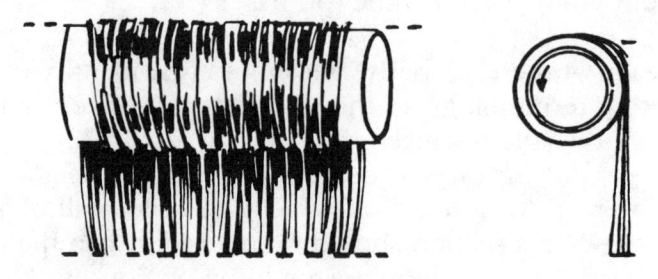

Fig. 6.16 Over-directed roller.

(c) Minimum volume is achieved by placing the roller so that it sits on the lower part of its base and is known as an under-directed roller. The base is equivalent to twice the diameter of the roller being used. Because the roller sits low on the base – as shown in Fig. 6.17 – less volume is achieved. This roller technique should be used whenever minimum lift is required.

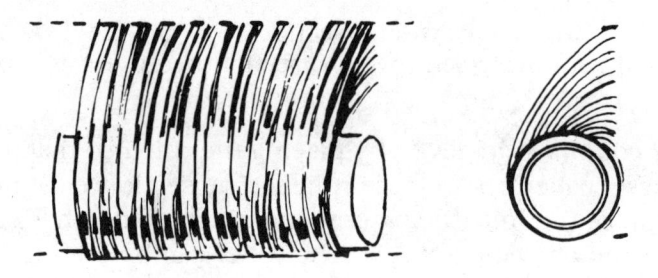

Fig. 6.17 Under-directed roller.

(d) Minimum volume on hairline is achieved by placing the roller so that it sits on the skin rather than on a base. Therefore, it can only be used on a hairline (i.e. nape, sides, front hairline). Because the roller does not sit on a base at all, it is known as being off-base, as shown in Fig. 6.18.

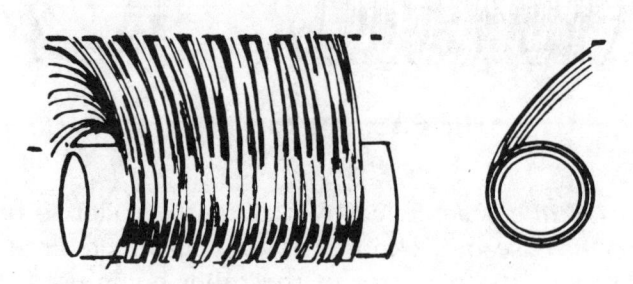

Fig. 6.18 Off-base roller.

(3) Roller direction

Apart from the stylist being able to control the degree of root volume that is achieved by using rollers, the hair is also directed by the careful positioning of the rollers. For example, a wave movement can be produced by the placing of rollers horizontally in opposite directions. This roller technique is on the same principle as reverse pincurling. This can be seen in Fig. 6.19, where one row is directed clockwise, while the following row is directed in an anticlockwise direction. Alternatively, rollers could be positioned to achieve a movement to one side, as shown in Fig. 6.20.

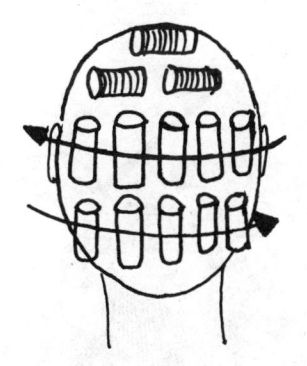

Fig. 6.19 Rollers are directed clockwise and anti-clockwise in alternate rows.

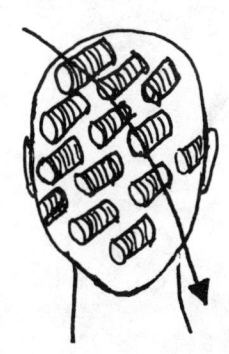

Fig. 6.20 Rollers are positioned to achieve movement to one side.

To produce a flick-up, the roller is wound in an upward direction, as shown in Fig. 6.21. The base size is made according to the amount of root lift that is required in the manner already explained.

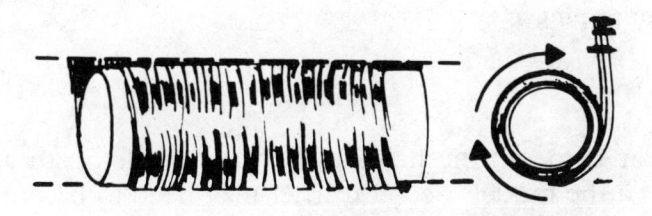

Fig. 6.21 Rolling technique to produce upward movement (flick-ups).

A summary of important points:

- Careful roller placement makes dressing the hair easier for the stylist and the client will find her style easier to manage at home.

150 Cutting and Styling: a salon handbook

- Ensure that the rollers are positioned in the direction of the intended style, using the correct roller technique to produce the desired degree of volume at the roots.
- Do not place rollers at right angles to the front hairline as this causes breaks in the dressing of the final style that are difficult to disguise.
- Wrap the hair evenly and cleanly around the roller to prevent buckled ends and to achieve enough tension on the hair. If the hair is wound too loosely around the roller it will produce a curl formation which is softer and looser than anticipated. The two diagrams in Fig. 6.22 show how you should hold the mesh straight and begin winding by folding the ends around the underside of the roller with either your thumb or index finger.

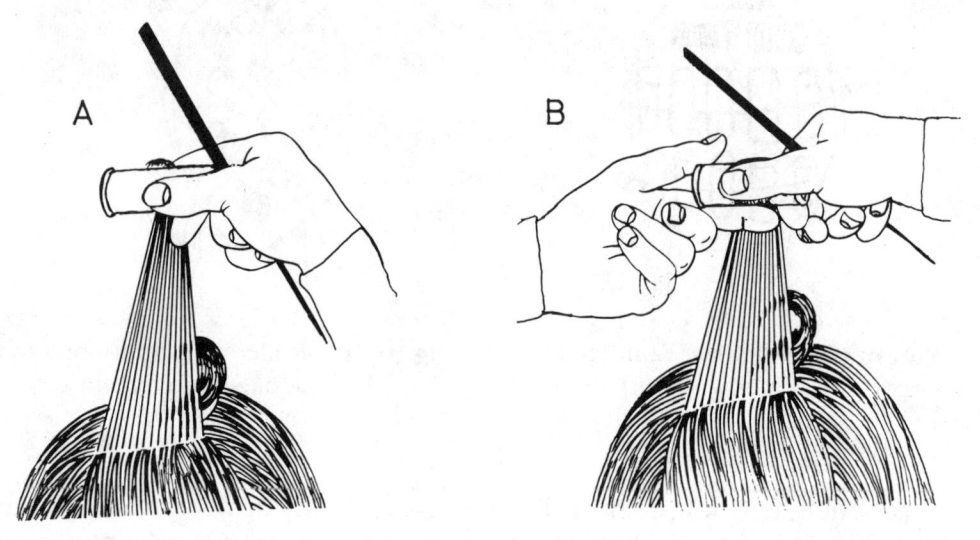

Fig. 6.22 A and B. Hold the mesh straight and begin winding by folding the ends around the underside of the roller with either your thumb or index finger.

Drying the hair

Once the hair is in pli, the hair can be dried underneath a hood drier. Depending on the model used, a hairnet may need to be positioned over the rollers and pincurls to ensure they are not disturbed by the airflow during drying. If a net is used, pads of cotton wool can be placed over the client's ears to protect them from the heat. Check that no pins or clips are placed in such a way as to cause discomfort to the client; make sure, for example, that they will not rest on the skin and cause burning once they become heated by the drier and that they are not digging into the client's skin. Try to remember to switch on the drier a few minutes before it is needed to give it time to reach a comfortable temperature.

Nothing is worse than having to sit under a cold drier on a winter's day. Make sure that your clients know how to adjust the temperature of the drier themselves, occasionally checking yourself that they are comfortable during the drying. Drying time will vary according to hair length and density, as well as the size of the rollers used. On average it is between 20–30 minutes. Highly bleached hair takes longer to dry than hair in good condition because it holds more moisture to begin with.

Checking that the hair is dry

The hair must be thoroughly dry before the rollers are removed. To check that this is so, remove a roller from the crown area and feel for any dampness by running your fingers from roots to points. Don't imagine that it will not matter if the hair is slightly damp. Because the hair is hygroscopic, the dampness will evaporate through the effect of body heat and be reabsorbed by the dry hair, causing the whole style to collapse. A roller at the back of the head should be checked in a similar way. If the hair is the slightest bit damp, replace the roller and continue with drying.

Removing the rollers

Once you are *sure* that the hair is dry, allow the hair a couple of minutes to cool before removing all the rollers and clips. This cooling period is essential before you proceed any further. If you should remove the rollers while the hair is hot, the hydrogen bonds could be broken by the heat and the desired curl pattern would be lost. It would be the equivalent of tonging the hair. If you are a little vague about what is being said here, go back to [6.1] and look at the sections comparing the chemistry of the cohesive and heat set.

If the hair is long, start removing the bottom rollers or clips at the back of the head first. This will prevent the hair from getting tangled as the rollers are removed. On shorter hair it makes no significant difference where the rollers or clips are taken out first.

Brushing the hair

Using a bristle or nylon tufted flat brush, brush the hair in the direction of the intended style to remove the roller marks and to make the hair manageable. At this stage, gloss creams should be applied to the hair if it is in need of nourishment or is full of static electricity. Continue brushing the hair and directing it into the shape of the intended style. By doing this, the stylist can see where backcombing or backbrushing will be necessary to achieve sufficient volume and height. Many stylists automatically begin backcombing every head of hair, without prior thought as to whether or not this is necessary. Some clients will prefer not to have their hair backcombed at all.

How do I deal with hair which has been set too tightly?

Sometimes you may find that you have misjudged the size of the roller that should have been used. To correct this, use a brush and hand drier to stretch the hair and so reduce the amount of curl. Be careful not to overdo this or you will end up having to replace the lost curl by using tongs. It is a safer practice to set hair too tightly than too loosely as it is quicker and easier to stretch out unwanted curl than it is to start tonging hair which is insufficiently curly.

When should backcombing be used?

Backcombing is a method of producing 'padding' in hair by pushing down the shorter hairs to the roots using the fine teeth of a comb. Backcombing also roughens the cuticle and so does cause damage to the hair. Sometimes the backcombing needs only to be done to give support at the roots of the hair, while other styles and hair types may require backcombing throughout the entire length of the hair. However much backcombing is put into hair, no backcombing should show in the final result.

How is hair backcombed?

A section of hair is held at right angles to the shape of the head, and this section should be no wider than the length of the comb or the depth of the teeth. If a section is too wide or deep, certain parts of the hair will be missed and the support you are aiming to produce in the hair will not be consistent. The comb is inserted into the hair about two-thirds of the way down its length and is pushed down towards the roots. The shorter hairs are pushed down to the roots of the hair, as shown in Fig. 6.23, and this is repeated several times until sufficient padding is achieved for the styling purpose. The hair mesh should be taken and held in a position which takes into account the direction of the intended style. This is called directional backcombing and ensures that the hair is being backcombed in the direction of the finished style. Try not to let the top side of the mesh get too messy; this can be avoided by not backcombing a mesh of hair which is narrower than the depth of the teeth on the comb. Once the hair is backcombed, it is gently combed or brushed into position with care not to drag out the backcombing. Ensure that all top hair is clean and that no backcombing shows. Backcombing is easier to carry out on hair which has been taper cut because there are more shorter hairs that can be pushed down than there would be with hair which has been club cut.

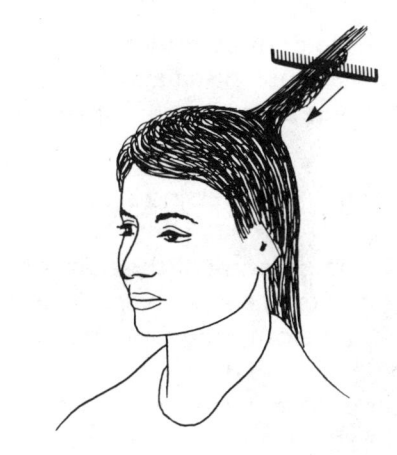

Fig. 6.23 Backcombing the underside of a section of hair.

When should backbrushing be used?

Backbrushing creates fullness in styles without the matted support of padding at the roots that backcombing produces. It is often better to use backbrushing on hair which is fine as backcombing is often difficult to clean and conceal. It is better on longer hair where a full curly look is wanted. Although not as supportive as backcombing, it is more easily removed from the hair.

How is hair backbrushed?

A bristle or nylon tufted flat brush can be used for backbrushing. The hair is held in larger quantities and is roughed up by the brush moving in a rolling action towards the points, as shown in Fig. 6.24. The shorter hairs are pushed downwards and the cuticle of the hair is roughened which increases the volume of the hair.

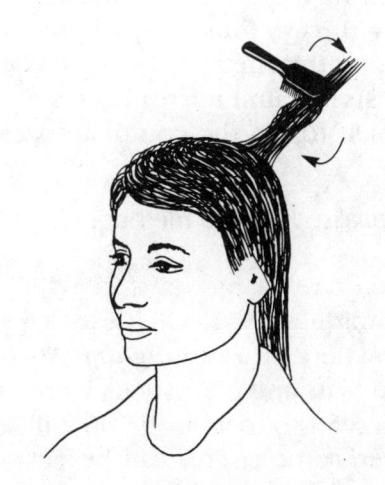

Fig. 6.24 Backbrushing – a slight turning action of the brush is used.

Backbrushing is a method of increasing the volume of the hair which produces more casual, and if desired, more tousled looks. Backcombing is used when a definite lift at the roots is required.

Completing the dressing

When the dressing of the hair is complete, check the hair from all angles to see the overall shape, balance and cleanness of the style. Use the mirror to check the front view and stand at the side of the client to see the profile shape. Stand so that your eyes are level with the back view (this will mean bending down) as stylists often forget to look to see how clean the nape hair looks. If both you and your client are satisfied with what you see, and are certain that no improvements can be made, the hair can be lightly sprayed with hair spray, if desired. Once hair has hair spray on it, it will create problems if you then try to rearrange it because the strands of hair will stick together.

See [6.6] for information on hairsprays, mousses and gels.

Using a back mirror

Clients are able to see their hair from the back if the stylist holds a mirror behind them to reflect an image which the client would not otherwise see onto the main styling mirror. When holding a back mirror, try not to move it around too quickly or you will not give the client enough time to see the back properly. Always check that back mirrors are kept clean and free from fingerprints and smears.

With very long hair, where it is not possible to show the client all of her hair by this method, turn the clients' chair around so that her back is facing the styling unit mirror. The client can then hold the back mirror in front of herself to see the complete back view reflected in the styling mirror.

Specialised setting methods

There are many ways in which hair can be set using various tools and techniques. We will describe the wrap round and the use of Molton Browners. In *Perming and Straightening – A Salon Handbook*, the use of Mad Mats and chopsticks were described as fashion perming techniques. If you refer to that book you will see how to wind to achieve the same results when setting. This can be very useful if you have a client who does not want an immediate permanent change in hair, as she can first try it out on a temporary basis!

Setting and Blow Drying

The wrap round

A wrap round is a setting method which can be used to straighten long wavy or curly hair temporarily.

Method

(1) Using very large rollers, place two on the crown using the on-base roller technique as in Fig. 6.25.

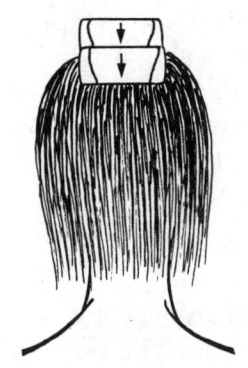

Fig. 6.25 Two rollers are placed on the crown using the on-base roller technique.

(2) Make a side parting and begin wrapping the hair around the head (the head acts like a large roller). Using a brush often helps the stylist to have greater control of the hair during wrapping and puts more tension on the hair, helping it to be stretched out more easily.

(3) The wrapping of the hair around the head continues until the head looks like Fig. 6.26, with all the hair sleekly stretched around the head. If possible, try not to use any clips on the hair to keep it in place as these will mark the hair, causing indentations on it. Instead, keep the hair wet and use a setting aid to bind the hair together.

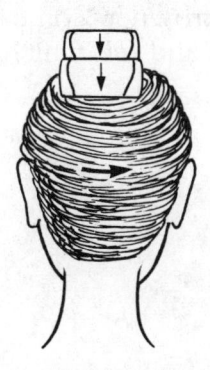

Fig. 6.26 The hair is wrapped around the head until it is sleekly stretched.

(4) The hair is protected by a setting net and dried under a hood drier, making sure that the net does not mark or disturb the wrapped hair when it is tied.

(5) Halfway through the drying time, some stylists re-wrap the hair in the opposite direction to prevent the roots from taking on one direction. This is a difficult procedure because the hair is semi-dry and tricky to control. This re-wrapping can be omitted.
(6) When the hair is dry, the rollers are removed and the wrap is undone and brushed. Because the hair will have dried to the direction in which it was wrapped, the stylist will now need to style the hair by blow drying it with a brush and hair drier. The hair is not re-damped, and small sections are taken to stretch and smooth the hair. When all the hair has been blow dried, the ends may require the use of tongs or a hot brush to achieve bend and body.

Molton Browners

Molton Browners are an alternative to using traditional setting rollers. They are not rigid, being made from cotton-covered wire and foam which is bent to hold in position, so do not require pins or clips. They can be used in a variety of ways to achieve tight curls, gentle waves on long hair, or bounce and body on shorter hair. Even waist-length hair can be set on Molton Browners which would be extremely tricky and time-consuming if conventional rollers were used.

Molton Browners should be used on clean, *dry* hair. The small amount of heat lost through the head is sufficient to aid the setting of dry hair. Additional heat from a hair drier can also be used to speed up the process. Molton Browners come in two sizes: pink which are half inch (1.25 cms) in diameter and red which are one inch (2.5 cms) in diameter.

Setting and Blow Drying 157

Method for creating deep waves in long hair

Use large sections of hair and the pink Molton Browners. First, twist the mesh of hair fairly tightly and then roll the twisted hair up along the Molton Browner. The Molton Browner is held in position by simply bending it in half, as can be seen in Fig. 6.27. A styling aid is sometimes applied to the hair (usually by spraying) at this point, but it can wet the hair too much as it will take a long time to dry while twisted. In the salon it is normal practice to put the head under a drier for between 10–15 minutes to help the hair take on the shape of the Molton Browners. The finished result can be seen in Fig. 6.28.

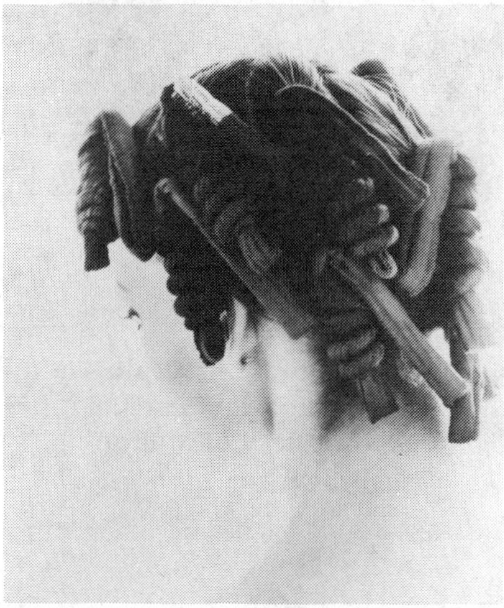

Fig. 6.27 Molton Browners are bent over to secure them in place on the head. The twisted hair can clearly be seen on the Molton Browners. (Courtesy of Molton Brown.)

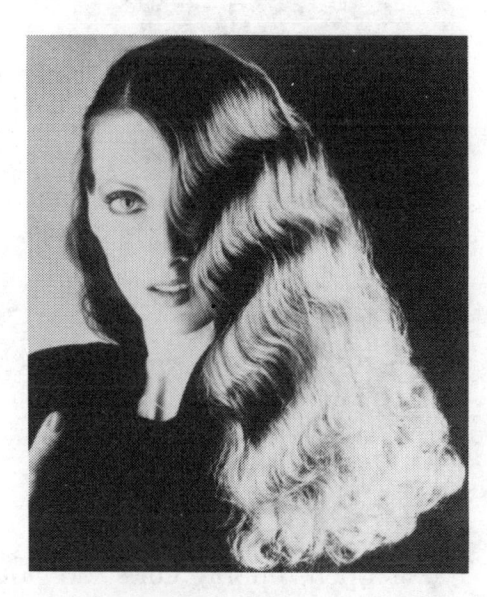

Fig. 6.28 Deep waves which were created using Molton Browners. (Courtesy of Molton Brown.)

Method for creating tight curls on long hair

The technique is exactly the same as before except that the sections need to be smaller. The completed set can be seen in Fig. 6.29, while the finished result can be seen in Fig. 6.30.

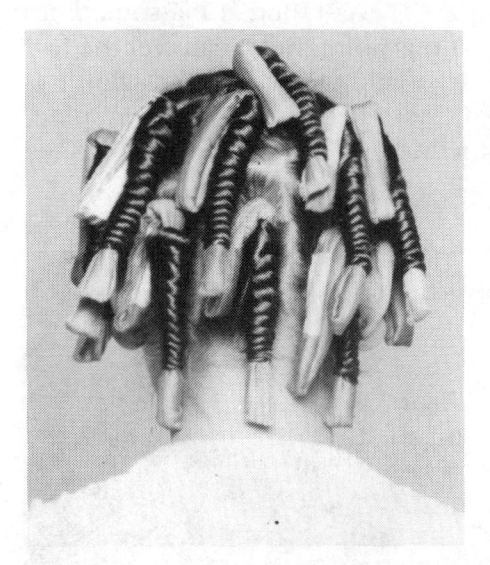

Fig. 6.29 Molton Browners wound to produce tight curls on long hair. (Courtesy of Molton Brown.)

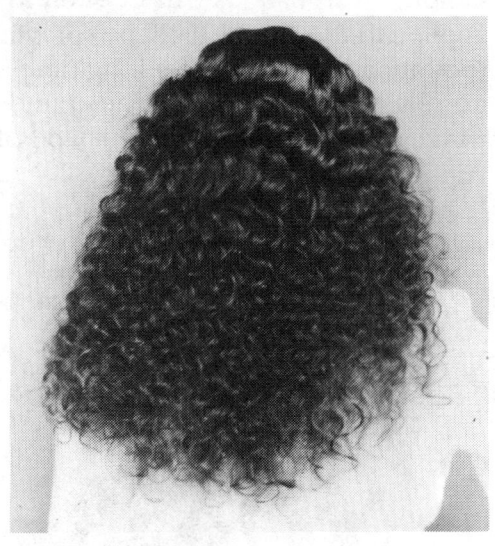

Fig. 6.30 The finished result is a mass of tight curls. (Courtesy of Molton Brown.)

For open, bubbly curls, do not twist the hair before rolling up. For setting medium length, layered and short hair, use the red Molton Browners, rolling the hair without twisting it first. By bending the sides of the Molton Browner forward the hair will be held in place.

6.5 Blow drying

Blow drying, or blow styling as it is also known, is the method of drying hair using a brush or the hands to mould and shape the hair into the intended shape and style. The hair needs to be cut into a good shape for it to fall into position easily; a bad haircut is difficult to disguise when it is blow dried.

Just as there are different techniques used for setting hair to achieve various effects, there are also different techniques of blow drying. A one length haircut would be blow dried using different techniques and tools than if you were blow drying a short, spiky look.

Principles for blow drying:

- The drier should always be kept moving to prevent burning the client's hair or scalp.
- The force and the temperature of the airflow should be adjusted according to the styling technique and type of hair you are working with. For example, fine hair will dry too quickly if a hot, fast drier setting is used. You will not have the time to create the required shape or direction before the hair dries.
- The root area of a mesh of hair should always be dried first before drying the middle lengths and ends. Lift at the roots cannot be achieved if they are not dried first.
- To increase the volume at the roots, over-direct the mesh of hair and direct the airflow in at the roots.
- The depth of the meshes to be dried should be no deeper than the equivalent of the diameter of the brush being used.
- Wherever you choose to begin drying the hair, it is essential that the mesh is completely dry before going on to another mesh. If you fail to dry a particular area, the moisture left in the hair will evaporate, causing the style to collapse.
- The drier should not be held too close to the hair or the heat will cause widespread and irreparable damage to the hair.
- When blow drying sleek styles such as bobs, the airflow should be directed downwards so that the cuticle is kept smooth (thus reflecting light and making the hair shiny) and the hair is kept as sleek as possible.
- The airflow should be carefully controlled at all times to prevent disturbance of the hair which has already been dried. It should not disturb the work of colleagues around you either!
- The hair is directed to the movement of the intended style, taking its direction from the roots.
- Only products intended for blow drying should be applied. Ordinary setting lotion will be sticky and will make the hair difficult to control.

Blow drying a one length shape

When drying a one length shape, such as a bob, you will be aiming to produce a sleek look with some bend on the points of the hair. A flat brush is the ideal tool for drying this type of style and the curve of the brush is what you will be using to produce the bend on the hair points.

160 Cutting and Styling: a salon handbook

Method using a flat brush

(1) Prepare hair with a styling aid if desired and make any partings that are required.
(2) Divide the hair into four sections (forehead to nape and across the top of the head from ear to ear) and secure each division with sectioning clips.
(3) Take a section, equivalent to the diameter of the brush you are using, ready for drying. This is shown in Fig. 6.31.

Fig. 6.31 Sections which are as wide as the diameter of the brush you are using are taken.

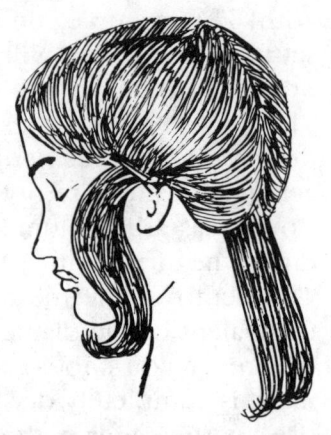

(4) Working with the hand drier in one hand and the brush in the other hand, place the brush underneath the mesh of hair at the roots. Keeping the tension on the mesh so that it is kept taut (without undue stress), direct the air flow in a downward movement onto the hair following the downward movement of the brush. Concentrate on drying the root area first, repeatedly introducing the brush to the roots once it has moved down the length of the hair. Repeat this movement until the hair is dry. Once the roots are dry, use the drier to style the middle lengths and ends, using the curve of the brush to achieve the bend on the hair points.
(5) Once the whole of the mesh is dry, take another section of hair (the same depth as the diameter of the brush) above the section you have dried. Dry this section of hair in the same manner as the previous one, ensuring that the root area is dried first. Continue in this manner until all of the back hair is dried.
(6) When you have completed the hair at the back, begin at the sides by taking horizontal meshes of hair on the underneath, gradually working upwards towards the parting or top hair. Figure 6.32 shows the final side being dried. Note how the brush is turned in the hand once it reaches the points of the hair, to utilise the curve of the brush and to create the bend on the points. The drier is held so that the airflow is directed downwards, keeping the hair smooth and sleek.

Fig. 6.32 The final side of the style being blow dried. The brush is turned in the hand once it reaches the points of the hair.

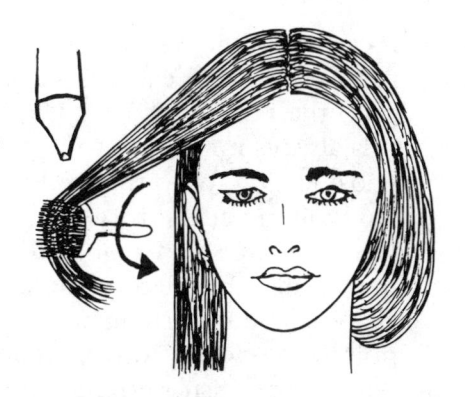

(7) To complete the blow dry the hair can be 'finger-pressed' to achieve optimum smoothness. This is done by taking meshes of the top, overlaying hair between the first two fingers and sliding them down the hair, followed by the airflow. This helps to flatten and smooth the cuticle even more, therefore achieving the maximum degree of shine on the hair.

(8) Once the blow dry is completed, you should always check that the hair is completely dry by feeling it with your hands. When the freshly dried hair is brushed, it should fall into the desired shape. If the ends do not turn under properly and tend to stick out when brushed, check that they are thoroughly dry; this will not occur if the hair is completely dry.

Blow drying using a circular brush

There are many different sizes of circular brushes, varying from about 1 cm in diameter to as much as 5 cms. The smaller the diameter of brush that is used, the greater the amount of movement and curl that will be achieved. It is important to remember that the smaller circular brushes should be carefully used as longer hair has a tendency to tangle with such brushes, especially if the hair is fine.

Large circular brushes can be used to shape one length hair shapes instead of flat brushes, but the smaller ones are mostly used on shorter lengths when curl is required.

Method

(1) Prepare hair with a styling aid if desired and comb the hair into its intended direction (that is, make any required parting and comb the hair according to the finished result).

(2) If the hair in the nape is long, it is recommended that the drying should commence in this area. Otherwise, the drying could begin wherever the stylist prefers. The important thing is that the blow dry

is carried out in a systematic way, using clean partings and correct size meshes, and that each mesh of hair is thoroughly dried before moving onto the next one.

(3) It is always important to dry the roots before the middle lengths and ends. Failing to do this will result in the stylist being unable to create any volume at the roots.

(4) Dry each mesh of hair and avoid disturbing the movement of curl until it has completely cooled as this will pull out the newly formed shape. When working with a circular brush, make sure that the hair points are cleanly wrapped around the bristles or you could end up with frizzy, distorted ends (that is, fish hooks).

(5) On completion of the blow dry, check that the hair is fully dry and look for any areas that require further styling. Also, check that the style is well-balanced in volume and that the hair is falling as intended. You may find it necessary to use tongs or a hot brush to achieve the desired degree of curl or movement, which is an acceptable practice. You should not rely on the tongs or hot brush to produce the style as your blow drying should have formed the hair into shape.

Blow drying using a vent brush

If you look at a vent brush, you will notice that the back of the brush has open spaces which allow the airflow from the drier to pass through. Also, the nylon bristles are of two different lengths. It is the venting on the back of the brush and these different length bristles that give the hair a casual, broken appearance when brushed. Therefore, blow drying with a vent brush is recommended when a textured, casual result is required. Vent brushes can also be used simply to brush through the hair after drying with a flat or circular brush, to break up the hair and create a softer, casual look.

Blow drying using the fingers

Sometimes, there is no substitute for the fingers to dry the hair into shape. The fingers are used to lift and direct the hair into the intended style, giving a softer and more casual appearance than using a brush. To create lots of volume and texture, as would be seen in spiky styles, place the palm of your hand flat onto the scalp and rotate it in a circular movement, directing the airflow onto this area. The hair will become matted, causing the hair to stand up. Sometimes, you may see stylists ask the client to bend her head forward so that the airflow can be directed underneath the hair at the nape. This helps to increase the body at the roots, making the hair stand out on the supporting hair underneath.

Scrunch drying

Scrunch drying is a method of blow drying using the hands which helps to increase curl and texture in hair which already has some natural movement. The root area should be dried first, perhaps asking the client to bend her head over to achieve maximum volume first. Then the middle lengths and ends are clasped tightly in the hands while directing heat on them from the drier.

Sections are not normally necessary when drying hair using this technique and quite large quantities of hair can be scrunched as opposed to small meshes. Do not be tempted to brush or comb the hair after scrunch drying as this would pull out the texture and movement you have created and all your hard work will be lost. Many stylists prefer to work with different diffuser attachments when drying hair using the scrunching technique.

Natural drying

There are certain looks that do not require to be shaped by a brush and hand drier. Instead they are combed or brushed into position and then allowed to dry naturally, perhaps occasionally lifting the hair with the fingers or an Afro comb. Such styles might be those which are permed and require no stretching by blow drying. Because it would be unreasonable to expect clients to sit in the salon waiting for their hair to dry as they would if they were at home, we use an additional source of heat to accelerate the process.

Perhaps the most popular means of drying hair naturally is by using heat provided from infra-red lamps in the form of some sort of accelerator, such as the Wella Climazon. The heat is dry and has no airflow to disturb the lie of the hair. Care must be taken that the light is not directed onto the client's face.

If you use a diffuser attachment on a hand hairdrier it will disperse the airflow and will cause little disturbance to the lie of the hair. Never allow the client to leave the salon with wet hair because it is possible to catch cold easily as the moisture evaporates.

Blow waving

The art of blow waving was developed as a technique during the nineteen-thirties, using a comb and hand drier to produce waves in the hair similar to those produced by finger waving. The comb is traditionally made from vulcanite to withstand the heat (though some modern plastic combs are heat-resistant). Blow waving should start at the front hairline, following the natural hairgrowth movement and direction. The wide teeth of the comb are used to hold the hair in the wave direction and the airflow is directed into the hair using a low power setting so that it does not blow the hair out of position. An important rule of blow waving is that the airflow is directed along the wave crest against the direction of the movement as shown in Fig. 6.33. Use a nozzle attachment to concentrate the airflow of the hairdrier.

Fig. 6.33 The air flow from the hairdrier is directed along the wave crest against the direction of the movement.

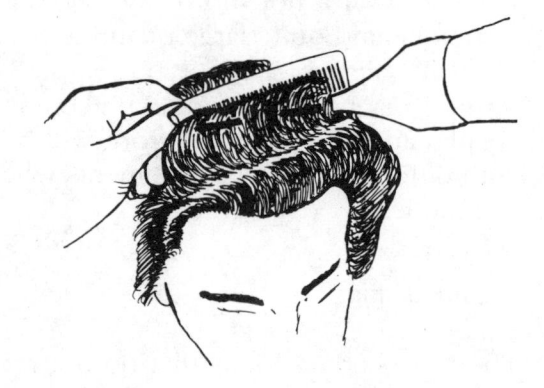

Relaxing over-curly hair

Blow drying using a brush can be used after the hair has been set on rollers to loosen the hair if it is too curly. The hair is not dampened, as it is the heat from the drier and the tension that you put on the hair that will relax the movement. When doing this, be careful to observe how the hair responds as it is very easy to over-relax the set, making it limp and lifeless. This technique is most frequently used after doing a wrap round to smooth out the hair.

6.6 Styling aids

At present these can be divided into setting lotions, hairsprays, mousses and gels. We will look at how they are used, and what they contain.

Setting lotions

These prevent the hair from drying out too quickly during setting and also help to prolong the life of the set by excluding atmospheric moisture from the hair shaft. There are historically two types of setting lotion, those older ones based on gums and the modern plastic setting lotions.

The gums were obtained when trees were damaged, as an exudation from the wounded bark. The two most well-known ones are gum tragacanth (Turkish) and gum karaya (Indian). When added to a solution of water and alcohol the gums form a sticky solution called a mucilage. Their use is now obsolete because they yielded dull, brittle films which crumbled into dust and became sticky in humid air because they were hygroscopic.

The modern setting lotions that you use in the salons contain plastic resins and polymers dissolved in a mixture of alcohol and water. The plastic resin is left as a flexible covering film on the hair when the water and alcohol have evaporated. They may contain resins or polymers such as polyvinyl pyrrolidone (PVP), polyvinyl acetate (PVA) or dimethyl-hydantoin formaldehyde resin (DMHF). Because PVP by itself is too hygroscopic, a copolymer of PVP and PVA is used in a ratio of 6:4; it is known as PVP-VA. To counteract any hardness of the plastic film, plasticisers are added. These are usually polyethyleneglycols and silicones. They make the film more flexible and water-resistant.

Setting lotions may also contain ingredients which are added to give the hair body and increased manageability. Plastic setting lotions intended for blow drying often contain silicone oils; these lessen friction, when brushing, by smoothing the cuticle of the hair. They also reduce heat damage as they are heat-resistant. Conditioners, such as protein hydrolysates, are often added. Some setting lotions containing acid dyes are available as temporary colours.

How is setting lotion applied?

The setting lotion usually comes in a small bottle holding between 10–20 mls. After shampooing, towel drying and disentangling the hair, a setting lotion is sprinkled (usually directly from the bottle) over the hair. To ensure that the lotion does not drip onto the client's face, one hand should be placed at the hairline while the lotion is applied. Placing the forefinger over the bottle opening will prevent the lotion from coming out too quickly. It is important that the lotion is evenly distributed throughout the hair and this is done by combing. The more alcohol in a setting lotion, the quicker it dries. Alcohol is a volatile liquid (i.e. it has a low boiling point) and evaporates off the hair quickly. Because of this it is also flammable, so store it away from sources of heat and do not use near naked flames.

How is a coloured setting lotion applied?

After preparing the hair as above, the lotion can either be applied by sprinkling, again as above, or with a tint brush. Some stylists prefer the brush application because the lotion can be more evenly applied in that way. Pour the lotion into a bowl and apply in the same way as for a tint (see *Colouring – A Salon Handbook*).

Hairsprays

Most salons use hairsprays which are supplied in aerosol cans. The actual spray is fine and makes an even application easier. They must be quick-drying and impart sufficient rigidity to the set to control it, without detracting from the natural sheen of the hair. They reached their height of popularity around 1970, and have fallen away since the advent of the mousse revolution of the 1980s. The resins used must be able to be shampooed off with ease yet not become powdery on brushing. The early ones contained shellac in alcohol. In 1948 this became available as an aerosol. Today it is the copolymers of PVP-VA which are most used. Other resins are used and about five new ones have been patented each year since the 1960s.

An aerosol is shown in Fig. 6.34. This one was developed by Goldwell and dispenses from the large can into a small, hand-held spray. The type that you are most familiar with is shown in Fig. 6.35. Once the spray button is depressed the hairspray is forced out of the can by the pressure of the propellant inside the can. (Some propellants (chlorofluorocarbons) were banned in the United States in 1979 because of their alleged damaging effect on the ozone layer above the earth, which acts as a shield against ultra-violet radiation. This led to the use of other propellants and hand pumps which are not as good as the original propellants for dispensing a fine spray.)

Because the propellant is volatile it forms a vapour at room temperature, which fills the space above the product in the can, the pressure of which drives out the hairspray (again, see Fig. 6.35). Never place aerosols near a source of heat or in direct sunlight on a hot day. The can can explode even after the contents have been used up. Never dispose of empty cans in fires.

Setting and Blow Drying **167**

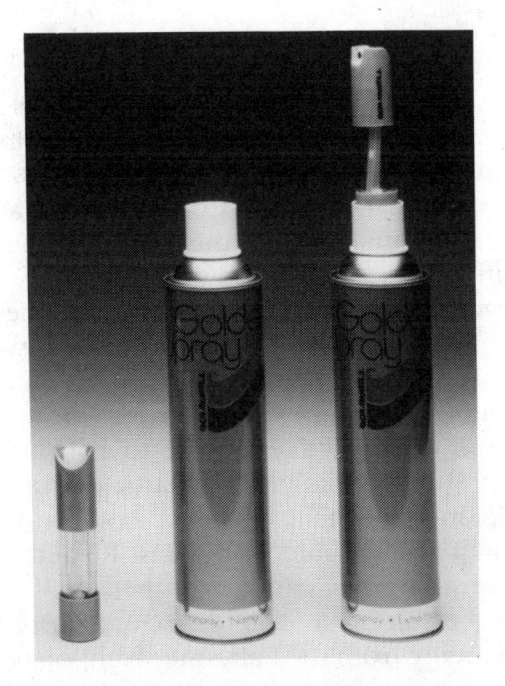

Fig. 6.34 This Goldwell hairspray has a small refillable spray which is filled by pressing it down onto the main container.

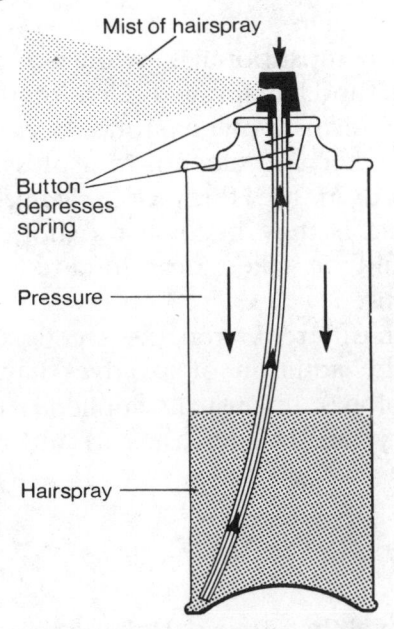

Fig. 6.35 A conventional aerosol can of hairspray. The nozzle of the button may become clogged from time to time.

Applying hairspray

The can should be held at a distance of approximately 30 cms (about a foot) away from the head and moved in a slight sweeping movement. The client's eyes, ears and neck should be protected by the stylist's free hand as hairspray can cause an allergic reaction on some skin and will irritate the eyes. If a client has soft contact lenses they should either take them out or keep the eyes tightly closed. This type of lens can be easily damaged by hairspray. If the spray is held too close to the hair the hair will become wet, separating into strands. Avoid inhaling hairspray, especially if you have a chest complaint such as asthma. Try to use hairspray in a well-ventilated area. Studies have not indicated any more serious problems, such as cancer, from prolonged exposure to hairsprays. Indeed, some studies have actually showed that PVP-VA particles can be eliminated from the lungs by the defence mechanisms of the body.

A word of warning about some hairsprays. Remember that if you use one containing glitter, the small particles of metal will react violently with hydrogen peroxide, resulting in hair damage. The glitter is often very difficult to remove totally from the hair; one shampoo may not be enough.

Mousses

Mousses are certainly the most popular styling aids of the 1980s. They are similar to setting lotions and hairsprays as far as ingredients are concerned, containing a solution of resins (polymers) and conditioning agents (silicone oils) in a mixture of water and alcohol in a pressurised container. The contents are dispensed in the form of a foam. Like hairsprays, the containers can explode if they become too hot, and the contents are flammable. Care should be taken near infra-red driers or even when smoking because of this.

Mousse is available in different strengths (see Fig. 6.36) to give increased holding power and the addition of azo-dyes has made it available in different temporary colours. It is usually applied to damp hair, although it may be applied to dry hair to increase curl and texture for scrunched looks.

How is mousse applied?

Always shake the can well before use. Holding the spout of the container downwards, apply mousse equivalent to the size of a small orange (more may be needed on long hair) to the palm of your hand. Spread the mousse between your hands and massage it through the hair. Comb the hair to ensure that the mousse is evenly distributed (this is especially important

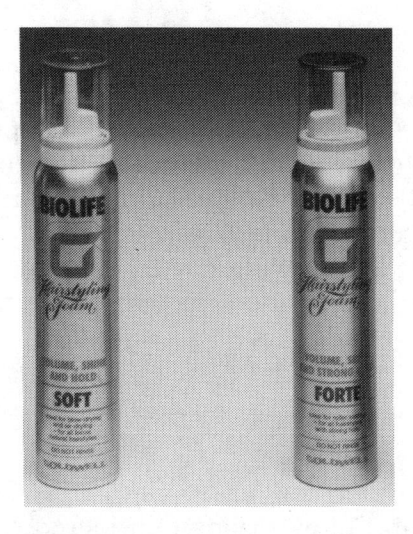

Fig. 6.36 Mousse is available in different strengths to give varying degrees of hold. (Courtesy of Goldwell.)

when applying a coloured mousse). Some stylists scoop the mousse from their hands onto a brush or comb to apply it to the hair.

Mousse can be revitalised the following day after application by running wet fingers or a wet brush against the direction of the finished look before final arrangement. Try different brands to see which one you like most. Some may be more greasy than others, depending on their exact formulations.

Gels

The popularity of hair gels has diminished with the advent of a broader range of mousses which are firmer holding. Originally, gels were preferred by many stylists because of their holding power. In hairdressing terms, two main types of gel are available: those which cannot be seen on the hair once it is dried, and those which create a wet-look, ideal for sleeked back styles. They can have added ingredients which make them flouresce or glow in the dark – ideal to be seen on a bike at night! Modern gels contain water-soluble plastic resins with a plasticiser to allow flexibility, although some preparations are deliberately made to make the hair stiff and unnatural-looking (punk styles, for example). Some clear gels are oil-in-water emulsions where tiny microscopic particles of oil are dispersed in water to give a less greasy feel than ordinary oil-in-water emulsions. These are sometimes called micro-gels.

How is gel applied?

After shampooing, when the hair is ready for styling, place a small blob of gel on your fingertips. Rub your hands together to spread the gel through the hair. Comb the hair to ensure that the gel is evenly distributed.

Gel may also be applied to the finished look by using the fingers to place the gel where a separated strand look is required, or for extra sleek looks. Gel can be revitalised the following day by running wet fingers or a wet brush through the hair against the direction of the finished look, before final arrangement.

6.7 Questions

1. Why are setting and blow drying considered temporary changes in the structure of hair?
2. Why is the degree of curl introduced into the hair slightly tighter than actually desired?
3. Would you consider setting to be a physical or a chemical change?
4. Why?
5. Why should setting be carried out on hair that is in good condition?
6. What bonds are broken during setting?
7. Why is stretching carried out on wet hair?
8. What is 'bound water' and what happens to it during the drying of hair?
9. Why does the dried hair stay in its new position?
10. What causes a set to drop?
11. What does 'hygroscopic' mean?
12. Explain the difference between alpha- and beta-keratin.
13. What is the difference between cohesive and heat setting?
14. How do you destroy a heat set?
15. Why is heat setting more damaging than a cohesive set?
16. Where does the word 'pli' originate?
17. What do the terms 'first and second pli' refer to when used correctly?
18. What are finger waves?
19. What effect does finger waving produce?
20. Draw a wave to show which part is the crest and which part is the trough.
21. What determines the height of the crest and the depth of the wave?
22. Why should you learn finger waving?
23. How do you prepare the hair for finger waving?
24. Making brief notes, describe how to carry out a finger wave.

Setting and Blow Drying 171

25 What are the main guidelines for finger waving?
If possible, carry out a finger wave on a block or a model.
26 What is pincurling?
27 How are pincurls secured in place?
28 What are the two main categories of pincurl?
29 What are the four main types of flat pincurls and when would you use each type?
30 Why is stem direction so important?
31 What are stand-up pincurls and when might you use them?
32 What is a combination pli?
33 What is roller setting?
34 Why should the hair be set in the direction of the finished style?
35 When should rollers not be used?
36 What are the three main principles behind the choice of roller techniques?
37 How do you judge correct roller size?
38 What are the four variations of root volume that can be achieved using rollers?
39 What do you understand by the term 'volume'?
40 How can different effects be achieved by roller direction?
41 Summarize the important points about setting using rollers.
42 What points should be kept in mind when drying the hair?
43 Why does bleached hair take longer to dry than hair in good condition?
44 Why is it important that all the hair should be dry before removing the rollers?
45 Why is a cooling period necessary before removing rollers?
46 How should hair that has been set too tightly be dealt with?
47 When and how should backcombing be used?
48 When and how should backbrushing be used?
49 How should you check the completed dressing?
50 Describe the ways that you could use a back mirror to check a client's hair if it were short or long.
51 Describe the wrap round.
52 How can you use Molton Browners to set hair?
53 What is blow drying?
54 What are the main principles of blow drying?
55 How do you blow dry a one length shape?
56 What are the differences between using a flat and a circular brush when blow drying?
57 What effect will a vent brush give when blow drying?
58 How do you blow dry using the fingers?
59 What is scrunch drying?

Cutting and Styling: a salon handbook

60 When would natural drying be used?
61 What effect does blow waving produce?
62 How can blow drying be used to relax over-curly hair?
63 What is the purpose of a setting lotion and what ingredients would you expect to find in a modern one?
64 What is 'mucilage' and why is its use now comparatively obsolete?
65 How are a colourless and a coloured setting lotion applied to the hair?
66 How would you apply a hairspray?
67 Are there any precautions that you would take when applying hairsprays?
68 How are mousse and hairspray similar?
69 How is a mousse applied?
70 What is a gel and how is it applied?

7
Treatments

The one area of real potential growth in salons, exclusively to do with hair, is *treatments*. Your clients enter the salon to have a service such as cut and blow dry, yet there may be other services that you can also offer them, depending on the condition of their hair and scalp. Few clients will have the quality of hair shown in Fig. 7.1

Just as fashions inevitably change, so do the ways in which people treat their hair. Recent statistics prove that women shampoo their hair far more

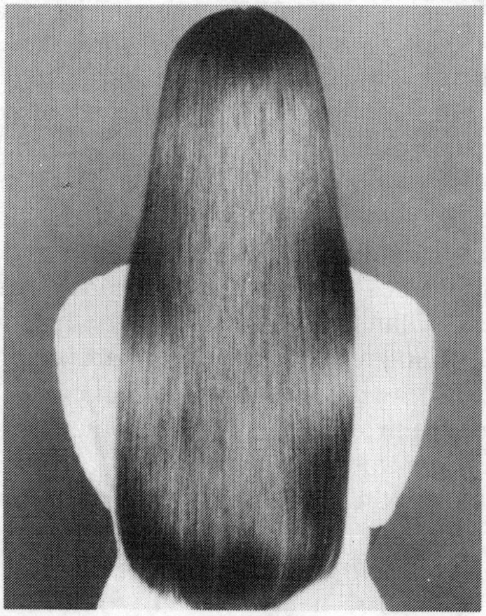

Fig. 7.1 A head of long hair in good condition. (Courtesy of Molton Brown.)

frequently today than in the past, a trend that men are also following. About 10 per cent shampoo their hair every day, while an incredible 65 per cent do so every two or three days. Of the 10 per cent that shampoo their hair every day, 44 per cent use a conditioner every time.

Surveys also definitely show that the public are concerned but ill-informed about their hair, and that is why *we*, the experts, should guide them. Those salons that provide a range of in-salon conditioners and treatments, backed up by a comprehensive retail range, will benefit financially from increased services and contented customers.

If we were absolutely candid about the services that we can offer in a salon, most of us would realise that some treatments and special shampoos do little to improve the hair and scalp, no matter what the rep or salesman says about his company's new wonder product. We are rather like the doctor giving harmless sugar pills or coloured liquids to patients, so that they will believe they are being treated and respond positively. Many of our hairdressing treatments, however, do make the hair look better and relax the client, making them feel more positive about themselves. When you feel good, you look good. The client should never be 'conned' – never told a product will permanently mend split ends or make their hair grow thicker, for example. If the product does not live up to its high expectations it will not be used again.

7.1 What's the problem?

Your clients come into the salon and ask for their usual hairdressing service – but have they got any other problems that you could help them with? First of all, what is their hair like? If it is greasy, how often does the client shampoo it? Many clients believe that it is wrong to shampoo their hair every day – so recommend a mild shampoo for them and tell them to wash it only once on each occasion (shampoos were dealt with in Chapter 4). What is the condition of the hair like? If the client uses heat on a regular basis, such as heated rollers or a hot brush, the hair will inevitably be in bad condition. Tell them what conditioners are available and how often they should be used. Suggest ways to achieve the same styling effect without creating as much damage. For a client with dry hair and scalp, suggest an oil treatment. If a client has dandruff, select a shampoo that will help to clear the condition. Suggest suitable treatment for other scaling conditions (see *Hygiene – A Salon Handbook*). Does the client have a tight scalp? The effect of a relieving massage can be nothing short of miraculous on some clients. They marvel at your insight to notice this! At the slightest sign of hair loss, sign your client up for a course of massage or high frequency, as well as conditioning treatments to boost the quality of the remaining hair. If you read *Hygiene – A Salon Handbook*, you will also be able to advise the client whom to see, if necessary.

7.2 Conditioners

Many conditioners are available, marketed by the major manufacturers as ranges of hair care products and usually in distinctive packaging. You will find it far easier to persuade clients to use a 'name' product which is nicely packaged and has already been made familiar through advertising. If you take on a range, demonstrations are often given on how to use them, with retail display stands and advertising literature. If clients buy a conditioner which they are pleased with they will be more likely to purchase shampoo and other items from the same range. An alternative to this is to have your own products made, bearing the salon name and *motif*. This is an excellent form of publicity for your salon, as it is something that usually only top salons do. Your salon can appear more successful than it really is! One major manufacturer supplies excellent products which are then repackaged by the salon.

What is a conditioner?

A conditioner is a special chemical which can be applied to the hair to help restore its strength, protect it against chemical damage and leave it shiny and manageable.

Why do we need conditioners?

The average scalp hair has an active growth period of three years (called the anagen phase of the hair growth cycle). This means that the hair will grow to approximately 45 cms (18 inches) in length if uncut. Throughout this period it will be subjected to the wind and weather, ultra-violet radiation from sunlight, brushing and combing (backcombing and brushing being particularly damaging), heat from drying and heated rollers, and possibly salt or chlorinated water when swimming in the sea or pools. All of these have a damaging effect, so it is little wonder that the hair frequently does not look its best. The cuticle bears the brunt of this. If you look at Fig. 7.2, you will see two photographs taken along different lengths of the same hair, showing longitudinal sections through the cuticle. In Fig. 7.2(a), which shows the cuticle of the hair at the opening of the follicle, the cuticle is intact. It is only a few days old, so has had little damage inflicted on it. However in Fig. 7.2(b), taken some 20 cms from the follicle opening,

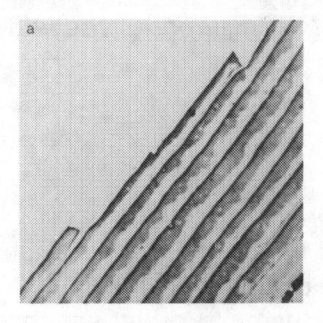

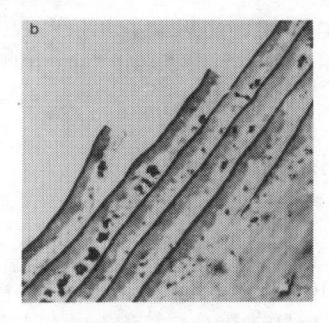

Fig. 7.2 Two photographs taken along different lengths of the same hair.
(a) The cuticle of the hair near the opening of the follicle.
(b) The cuticle 20 cms from the follicle opening. You can clearly see the effects of age on the cuticle. (Courtesy of Wella Ltd.)

the edges of the cuticle are raised and there are tiny vacuoles which are visible as dark 'spots'. The edges of the overlapping scales have become irregular and jagged, flaking outwards and causing tangling with other hairs. The roughened surface gives rise to resistance against combing, a build-up in static electricity and a resultant difficulty in keeping the hair under control. As the cuticle wears away, sometimes becoming almost non-existent, split ends form.

So far we have described the ravages of physical abuse, without the added damage caused by hairdressing chemicals. Modern shampoos degrease the hair shaft, while the hydrogen peroxide used in bleaching and tinting weakens the fibres of the cortex with a resultant loss in elasticity. The chemicals found in perm lotions and straighteners attack the disulphide and peptide bonds of keratin, and although some of this is repaired by neutralisation, some residual damage is inevitable, even with correct chemical techniques. When the hair is overprocessed the results can be disastrous; the hair can break off or feel like straw!

What types of conditioner are there?

Today's conditioners are the sophisticated scientific versions of the earlier ones which were based mostly on vegetable oils and eggs. They may be formulated to be applied either before or after a hairdressing procedure (a pre- or post-treatment). To a great extent conditioners must be substantive to hair – that is, be attracted to it. Because keratin is anionic – that is, has negative charges – this is easily achieved by having a conditioner with positive charges. The more damaged or porous a head of hair is, the more conditioner it can attract and hold. The first conditioners introduced in 1945 were based on cationic (positively charged) compounds. But, a word of warning! Because cationic compounds are positive they are incompatible (i.e. they cancel out each other) with anionic ones such as the majority of shampoos. Therefore you should never use a shampoo after a cationic conditioner. Conditioners can be grouped into three main categories:

(1) oils;
(2) acids;
(3) substantive.

(1) Oils
Since antiquity oils have been used to lubricate and add lustre to the hair. They have a high refractive index. (The refractive index is a measure of the degree to which light is bent on passing from one substance to another, so substances like diamond which have high refractive indexes reflect light more.) Therefore, oils will give the hair lustre. A thin layer of oil will also reduce friction when the hair is combed or brushed and help the hair to retain moisture. Oils must be used sparingly, to avoid excessive greasiness. A small amount should be spread over a large area of hair or the excess should be rinsed out if more is applied. The oil is usually in the form of a dilute oil-in-water emulsion and may be lanolin or a synthetic product, made to resemble sebum. Silicones have a good conditioning effect on the hair and leave behind a film of polymer after rinsing. They are added to many products which need built-in conditioners to prevent damage. Hot oil treatments are considered in [7.3].

(2) Acids
Traditionally, weak acid rinses were used to remove soap scum, neutralise any excess alkali left on the hair after a chemical processing treatment and to impart a sheen to the hair. Weak organic acids such as acetic acid (vinegar) and citric acid (lemon juice) were used to close the cuticle. Their main use today is after chemical processing, soap scum being a thing of the past as shampoos today are soapless. The preferred acid today is ascorbic acid (also known as vitamin C), because it is also an antioxidant, helping to stop the action of hydrogen peroxide after bleaching, perming and tinting. Rupture of peptide bonds by hydrogen peroxide or ammonium thioglycollate produces water-soluble products which would be lost on subsequent shampooing, thus weakening the hair fibres. Acids cause these soluble products to precipitate or solidify, thus preventing their loss.

(3) Substantive
This group of conditioners includes cationic detergents and protein hydrolysates. There are other chemicals with conditioning properties, such as PVP and non-ionic detergents which are added to hairdressing products.

The best known cationic conditioner is cetrimide (chemically a quaternary ammonium compound), its positive charge being attracted to the negatively charged hair. It reduces static, softens the hair, and makes it easier to comb. The antistatic effect is due to the retention of moisture. If you refer back to shampoos in Chapter 4, you will remember that cetrimide can be extremely damaging to the eyes.

The so-called proteins are actually mixtures of the breakdown products of proteins (polypeptide chains, peptides and amino acids), which have been prepared by hydrolysing protein. (Hydrolysis is the breakdown of a substance by its reaction with water.) The protein hydrolysates thus formed are attracted to the hair in much the same way as salt linkages (similar to opposite charges); basic groups are attracted to acid groups and vice versa. As hair damaged by chemical processes contains more of these free groups, such hair will attract more protein than undamaged hair. There is no real need to have exotic sources of protein such as placenta, but it certainly sounds impressive! If a conditioner contains hydrolysed keratin it has usually come from sources such as hoofs and horns, while if it is human keratin it will have been obtained from old hair cuttings.

A number of experiments have been conducted with protein conditioners to prove that they do combine with the hair. These include the use of radioactive labels, amino acid analysis and staining. These techniques have been shown to protect damaged hair during bleaching and perming. Scientific experiments have shown that little damage was caused to protein-treated hair while untreated hair suffered extensive damage. It is recommended, therefore, that protein hydrolysates should be used before chemical treatment. They have also been shown to help make split ends cling together by electrostatic attraction.

Hair restructurants or strengtheners

As their name implies, these are products which claim to help rebuild some of the damage that the hair may have suffered. They are usually individually packed and because of their ingredients cannot be stored after opening. They are applied to towel-dried hair after shampooing. The ingredients should be mixed as required and sprinkled over the hair before combing through. They normally contain a setting agent and are not rinsed out of the hair after application. the restructurant contains chemicals which help to establish new cross-links between the hair fibres. They usually contain an acid catalyst which forms a hair strengthening resin within the hair fibres, making the hair virtually insoluble in water.

How are conditioners applied?

This depends to some extent on the manufacturer and the purpose of the conditioner. Some are used to protect the hair before chemical processing (see *Perming and Straightening – A Salon Handbook*) while others are used to repair damage, sometimes on a regular basis after shampooing the hair. In the latter case, towel-dry the hair to remove excessive moisture, or the conditioner will be diluted. Conditioners can be applied with a tint brush, as shown in Fig. 7.3, in much the same way as you would apply a

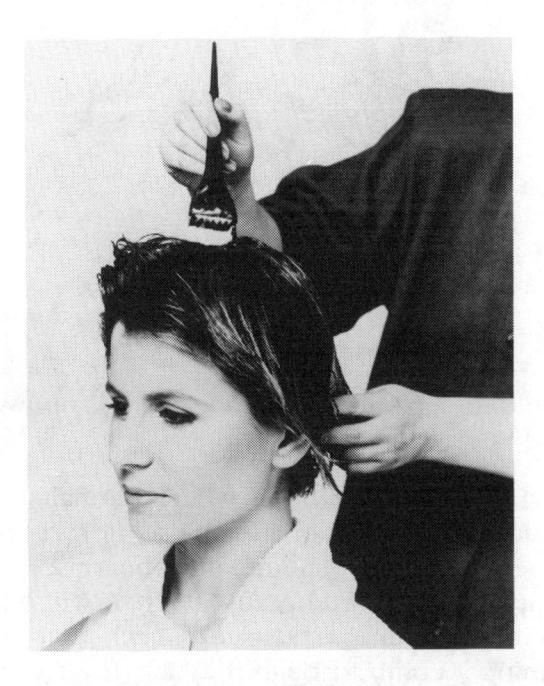

Fig. 7.3 Applying conditioner with a tint brush. (Courtesy of Trevor Sorbie.)

tint. Alternatively, they can be applied directly with the hands. Pour the conditioner into the palm of your hand and then distribute between your hands. Smooth your hands through the hair, distributing the conditioner through the hair. Gently massage the product through the hair, ensuring that all the hair is treated with the conditioner. Use your fingers like a comb to disentangle the hair or alternatively use a wide-toothed comb to remove tangles. The application may look like that in Fig. 7.4.

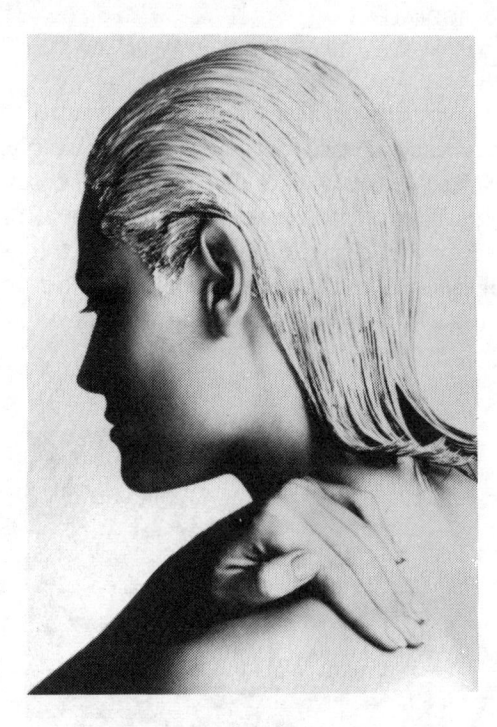

Fig. 7.4 Completed application of conditioner. (Courtesy of L'Oréal.)

The product will be taken up more where the hair is most damaged. Leave the conditioner on the hair as long as is recommended by the manufacturer. The conditioner should then be rinsed out of the hair, making sure that it is all removed because the hair will otherwise become greasy, flop and be difficult to manage. Check that rinsing has been thorough by running a comb through the hair. If a foam appears on the comb, there is still conditioner present which needs to be rinsed off.

Some conditioners will require heat to aid penetration into the cortex. This can be supplied by using hot towels (to form a turban as shown in Fig. 7.5), steamers, accelerators (Climazon) or hood driers (place a plastic cap over the client's hair). Remember to switch on steamers and hairdriers before they are needed so that they warm up. If you use hot towels they will have to be replaced as they cool down. A hot towel is made by soaking it in very hot water and squeezing it out; however, it should not be so hot as to scald the client!

What are surface and penetrating conditioners?

Many hairdressers refer to the conditioners that work on the cuticle alone as 'surface conditioners'. These will remove tangles from hair by

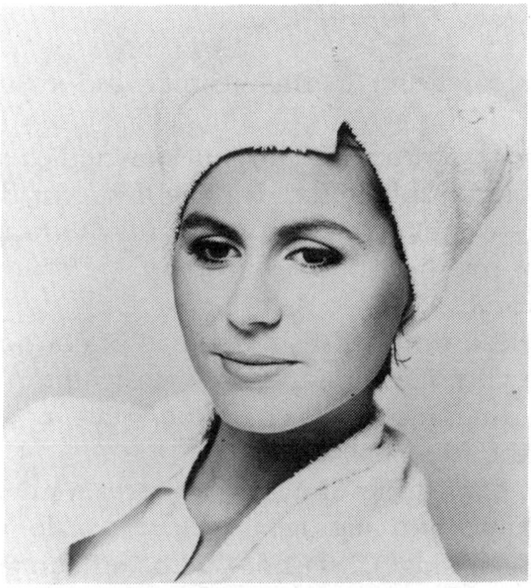

Fig. 7.5 Hot towels are applied in the form of a turban. (Courtesy of Trevor Sorbie.)

smoothing down the cuticle and are usually very quick-acting, so do not need to be left on the hair long. The penetrating conditioners are intended to help repair the cortex and may take longer to work than surface conditioners. You should be able to classify conditioners into these two groups (if you really want to!) by what the manufacturers claim they can do or if heat needs to be applied to aid penetration.

In general, surface conditioners will be those that contain natural (lanolin) or synthetic (silicone) oils to coat and lubricate the cuticle or acids to close it. Penetrating conditioners may also be referred to as reconditioning creams or restructurants. They contain protein fragments, quaternary ammonium compounds and synthetic chemicals, often containing urea.

7.3 Oil treatments

Vegetable oils, such as olive, avocado and almond oils, have traditionally been used in hot oil treatments on clients with dry hair and scalps. These have largely fallen into disuse and have been replaced by oil shampoos and cetrimide rinses. They are difficult to remove from the hair but could be asked for by some clients who are worried about dry scalps. The treatment can be obtained in individual application bottles, which can look better to the client than getting out a huge container of oil!

How do I carry out an oil treatment?

(1) Check the level of water in the steamer and switch on for a few minutes.
(2) Place the steamer over the head of your gowned client and make sure that they are comfortable before leaving them for five minutes.
(3) Heat the oil in a double container (this utilises a water jacket so that the oil does not overheat or get burnt).
(4) Remove the steamer.
(5) Using either a clean tinting brush, or a pad of cotton wool, apply the oil to the scalp and, if necessary, right up to the points of the hair. Make small partings about 1 cm wide, starting in the nape and proceeding to the front hairline.
(6) Place the client back under the steamer for ten minutes.
(7) Remove the steamer and massage the client's scalp (see [7.4] for a full explanation of massage), starting with effleurage, going on to petrissage and finishing off with more effleurage.
(8) After the massage has been completed, apply some soapless shampoo directly onto the client's scalp without any water. Massage the shampoo thoroughly into the hair, as this will help to emulsify or break up the oil. Using water straight away is likely to help spread the oil over the hair shaft, making it more difficult to remove. Rinse off with hot water and repeat again. The hair is free from oil when it is 'squeaky' clean.

Do not give an oil treatment before any chemical processing is to be carried out or it could create a barrier.

7.4 Massage

Massage is best described as the physical manipulation of the soft outer tissues of the body. It is one of the most ancient ways to reduce pain and tension. People who can give a good massage are often referred to as having 'magic hands'!

What effects has a massage on the scalp?

There has been some controversy in the past about the real physiological value of massage. Basically it stimulates the scalp. The blood vessels dilate and the scalp becomes redder in colour (this redness of the skin is referred to as a hyperaemia), giving the benefit of an increased blood supply to the papillae of the hair follicles (this provides extra oxygen, glucose and amino acids for cell growth). The drainage of blood is also increased from the scalp, which helps remove waste respiratory gases such as carbon dioxide. The lymphatic system is also stimulated which helps with the removal of waste products. The mechanical stimulation of the nerve supply increases the secretion of sweat from the eccrine sweat glands, again increasing the removal of waste products. Stimulation of the arrector pili muscle attached to each hair follicle causes the hair to rise and increases the rupture of fat cells. This indirectly stimulates the constriction of the sebaceous glands which secrete more sebum (hence massage can be good for a dry scalp). Besides these physiological benefits, the massage can decrease tension and pain, making the subject more relaxed.

Contra-indications to massage

If the client has an infectious condition such as impetigo or ringworm a massage should not be given. The scalp should be checked for head lice; do not proceed if these are present. If a client has broken skin, check for reasons such as infections and do not proceed as you might open up the breaks further. If the scalp is inflamed (red and tender-looking) do not proceed. Never massage if a client has just been on a sunbed or is sunburnt or they might pass out on you! Do not massage a client who has low blood pressure or any kind of heart or circulatory disorder; ask about this or you may cause your client to blackout. Massage should not be performed on a client with an above normal temperature, as might occur with flu or a fever.

How should you prepare yourself to give a massage?

Wash your hands and thoroughly dry them before beginning the massage. If your hands are very cold, your client will appreciate your doing this in hot water to warm them up! Stand behind the client with your weight evenly distributed on both feet. A word of warning! Your nails should not be too long or you could scratch your client's scalp.

How should you prepare the client for a massage?

You should already have checked the client's scalp for infections, etc. It is essential that the client is completely relaxed before the massage starts. Nervous clients should be calmed down and told how much they will enjoy it! Seat the client in an upright but comfortable position. Loosen any constrictive clothing around the neck. The hair should be free from tangles. Since the threshold of discomfort and pain varies from person to person, you should question the client frequently about any uncomfortable sensations.

What are the techniques of hand massage?

There are five basic techniques of hand massage:

(1) effleurage;
(2) petrissage;
(3) tapotement;
(4) friction;
(5) vibration.

(1) Effleurage
This is a stroking movement which should be used to begin and end a massage. With the fingers together, mould your hands to the head. Stroke the scalp from the frontal hairline right back to the base of the occipital bone (almost to the top of the shoulder blades) in one continuous movement. Be careful not to pull the hair. Try to build up an even, firm pressure with these stroking movements. Cover the left and right sides of the head, always stroking from the front hairline towards the nape. Many people will tell you that you should use both hands together, but it does not matter if you make alternate strokes with each hand. If it is your first massage, do it whichever way feels most natural to you. This type of massage should be continued for at least a couple of minutes and will soothe and relax your client. If you tell your client that you can already feel her scalp loosening she will be very happy!

(2) Petrissage
This is described as a kneading movement, because the scalp is kneaded in almost the same way a baker kneads dough. The pads of the fingers are placed a little apart on the scalp, one hand on each side of the scalp. While exerting light pressure, move the scalp with your finger tips in a circular direction. You should be moving the client's scalp and not your fingertips! If you move your fingers against the skin and hair you might damage the hair. Use your hands to support the client's head. Do not be shocked if the client falls asleep during the massage because she is so relaxed; it is a compliment to your skill. If you look at Fig. 7.6, you will see how the hairdresser is standing behind the client, making these kneading movements. Keep this massage up for 5–10 minutes. You actually will notice the scalp loosening with this movement, which breaks down the fat and increases the removal of waste products. If you do not proceed to the next movement, finish the massage off with a few minutes of effleurage. Gradually decrease the pressure of your stroking movements as you massage again for a couple of minutes.

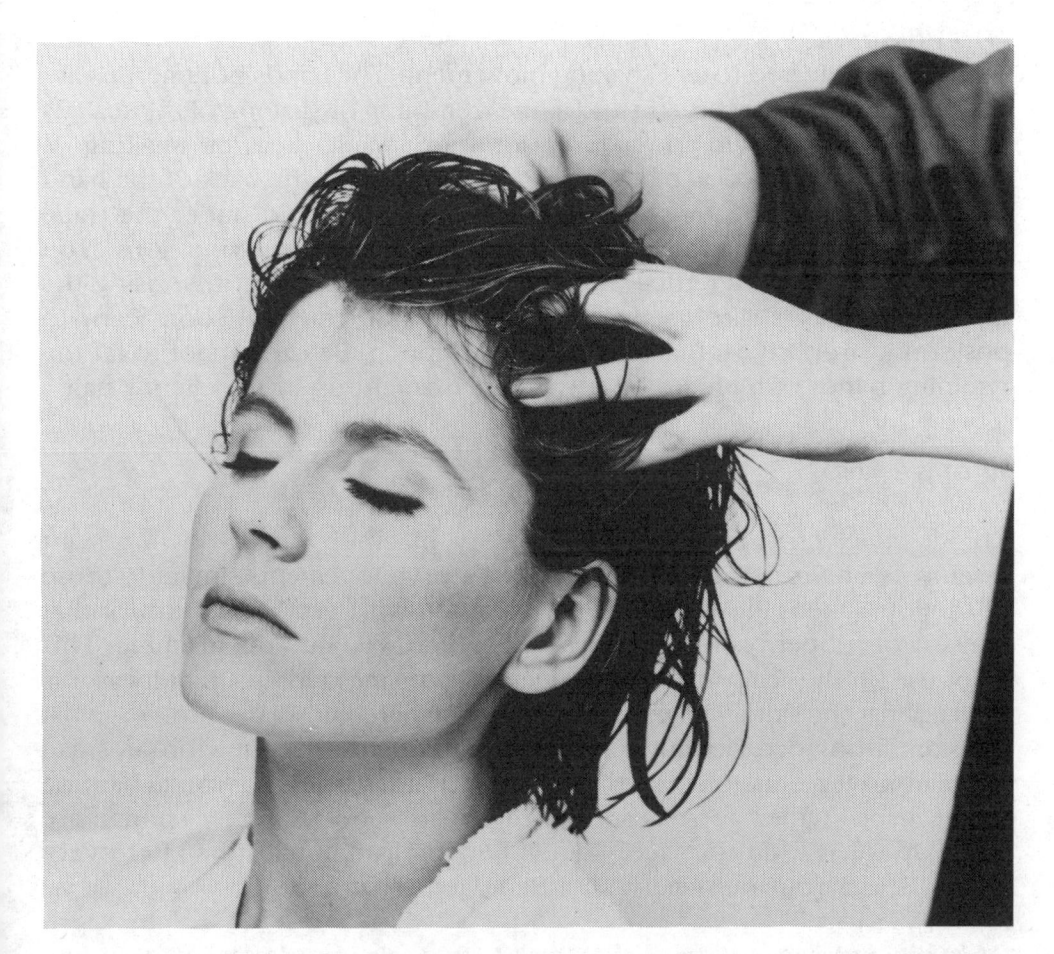

Fig. 7.6 Petrissage is used to loosen the scalp of the client. Notice that the stylist stands behind the client. (Courtesy of Trevor Sorbie.)

(3) Tapotement
This means percussion or tapping. In hairdressing this is carried out with the tips of the fingers. The tapping should be as quick as possible and it quickly gets tiring! It is very difficult to achieve the proper intensity. This movement is not particularly effective on the scalp. On the body the same term is used to describe quick 'chopping' with the sides of the hands.

(4) Friction
This type of massage refers to a small deep movement with great pressure, performed in a circular direction with the thumb and fingertips (some examining bodies wrongly refer to it as a 'light rubbing' movement with the fingertips, the friction thus created producing heat). Surface rubbing of the skin is likely to produce irritation and possible inflammatory reactions, as well as hair breakage. The skin must be moved against the skull below.

(5) Vibration

This can be referred to as a shaking movement. The hands or fingertips are placed firmly against the skin and a fine trembling or shaking of the scalp is performed. Light vibrations are soothing while heavier shaking is stimulating. An electrical machine can be strapped to the back of the hand to make this type of massage easier. The machine, sold under the trade name of 'Stimulux' can be set to provide weak or strong vibrations. You simply place your fingertips onto the client's scalp. When first using the machine it may shake itself off your hand but you will soon learn to position it properly so that this does not happen. Be careful not to let the retaining bands, which are often wire, get caught up in the client's hair.

What is a vibro?

This is an electrically operated vibratory machine which on first sight resembles a hairdrier. It can produce vibratory movements similar to those of friction. One is illustrated in Fig. 7.7, fitted with a spiked applicator that consists of rubber prongs on a base that is screwed into the machine. This is for use on the scalp and the surface of the prongs vibrates rapidly as it is held against the skin. The machine should be held lightly but firmly against the skin, lifting occasionally to prevent hair tangles. Use the vibro in small circular movements to cover the scalp, or in lines from the frontal hairline to the nape. Other applicators which consist of soft rubber sponge are available for use on the face. Remember to clean applicators after every client. Finish your massage with effleurage by hand.

After any massage, allow clients to rest for a few minutes before standing up or they may feel dizzy or faint. Wash your own hands.

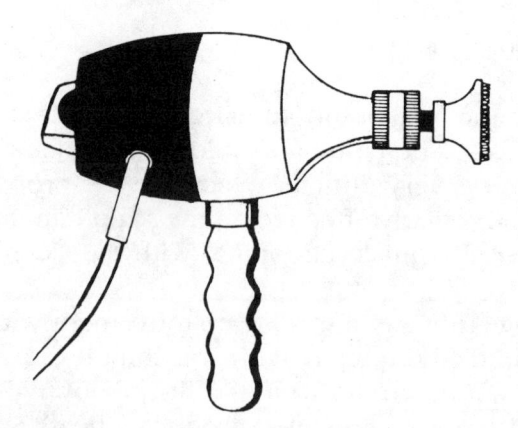

Fig. 7.7 An electric vibro machine fitted with an applicator.

7.5 High frequency

This is still taught in most colleges, but has become a rare service in the majority of salons. The high frequency machine produces a high voltage with a low current, so is safe (when used properly); car batteries have a low voltage but a high current, so can give a nasty shock. The machine is usually seen as a small portable black box, like the one illustrated in Fig. 7.8. It is plugged into the mains and the electrodes are fitted into a holder.

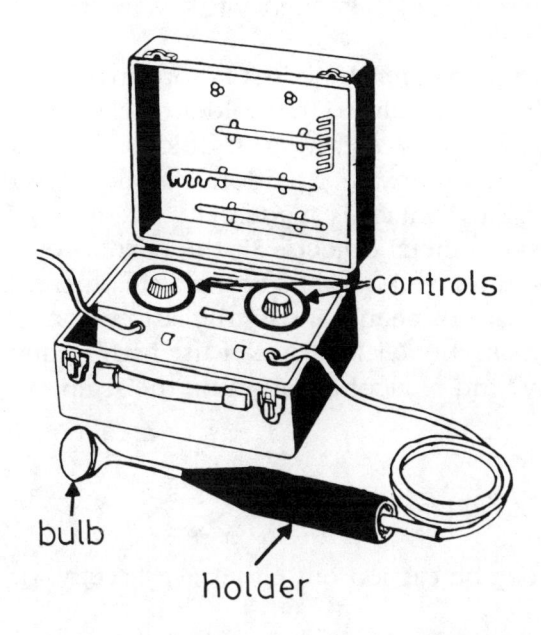

Fig. 7.8 A high frequency machine complete with electrodes in the box.

Why give high frequency treatments?

High frequency treatments will stimulate the scalp and when used frequently will benefit hair loss conditions. It can induce hyperaemia (redness of skin due to increased blood flow) which increases the supply of nutrients to hair follicles. Do not tell your client that it will stop hair loss; it won't, but it may help slow it down. The gas ozone is produced during high frequency and this has a slight antiseptic action. Ozone is a form of oxygen which contains three atoms of oxygen rather than two, the normal form we breathe in. You will be able to smell the ozone, which might remind you of the seaside because this is another area where ozone is produced. This is one reason why the sea air is so 'bracing'. Like hand massage, high frequency is relaxing and can have a positive psychological effect if carried out correctly.

Are there any contra-indications to giving high frequency?

Yes. It should never be given to anyone who has an infectious skin condition such as ringworm or impetigo, head lice or inflamed skin. Also ask your clients if they have any kind of heart trouble, including whether they have a pacemaker; if so, do not give treatment. Never give treatment to pregnant women or anyone on medication.

How do I prepare to give high frequency to my client?

Check the high frequency machine first before any treatment, checking for any damaged cables or cracks to the holder or glass electrodes. Any loose jewellery, such as bracelets or earrings should be removed from both your client and yourself, otherwise irritation can be caused by sparking of electricity when skin contact is made. The client should also be placed away from water and metal objects. Sit the clients comfortably in a chair and try to get them relaxed before starting a treatment. Electrodes should be cleaned if this has not been done by the last person to use the machine. Remove tangles from the *dry* hair. Never use high frequency if a client has recently used any kind of alcohol lotion on the scalp, or the vapour could ignite!

How do I carry out high frequency?

High frequency can be carried out either (1) directly, or (2) indirectly:

(1) The direct method
This is carried out by inserting the glass electrodes into the holder and drawing them through the hair. The electrodes should be inserted with the current turned off. They should fit snugly into the holder. Never force them in or out of the holder or the glass could break. If you look at the lid of the high frequency box in Fig. 7.8 you will see the electrodes held by clips. From top to bottom, you see the glass bulb, rake and comb, below which is the metal saturator rod. Use the bulb on bald areas or areas with little hair and the rake and comb on the normal scalp hair. Grip the holder in one hand, turn the current on low to start with and place one finger of your free hand onto the top of the glass electrode you are using. This is illustrated in Fig. 7.9 with a rake. Do not remove your finger until the electrode is in contact with the client. This prevents sudden sparking, which may be uncomfortable for the client, between the hair and skin. Do this every time the electrode is removed from scalp contact before reapplying. Use the bulb in a small circular movement for between 2–5

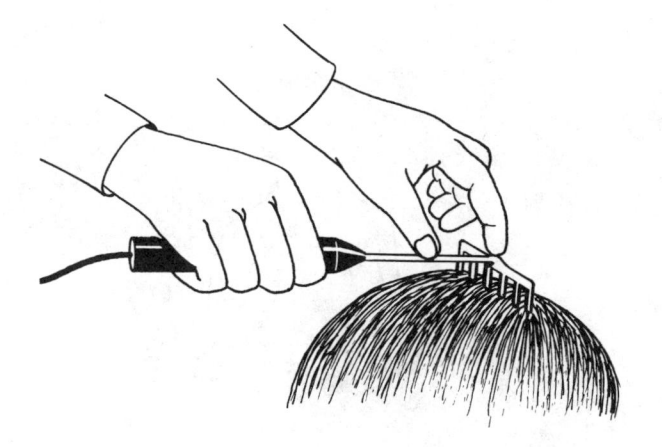

Fig. 7.9 The tip of the index finger should be kept on the electrode until it is in contact with the head.

minutes. As the client gets used to the treatment you will be able to increase the current by turning one of the dials on the machine. Do not be frightened by the violet light that is produced in the glass electrodes. When using the rake or comb be careful not to get them tangled in the hair. Starting at the front hairline, gradually work towards the nape by drawing the electrode through the hair. Be careful to avoid lifting the electrode clear of the scalp or hair, otherwise painful sparking may result. A treatment should last no longer than about ten minutes. The direct method of application may be combined with the indirect method to wind up a treatment.

(2) The indirect method

This is carried out by inserting the metal saturating bar into the holder and asking the client to hold it, one hand on the metal bar and the other on the holder, or as shown in Fig. 7.10. Emphasise to clients that they should not release their hands as they will get a sudden shock. The client will not feel anything until you place your hands onto the scalp. As the fingers touch the skin the current flows from the bar through the client's body to the point of contact with the client – i.e. your fingers. Carry out a gentle massage. With practice you will be able to create a slight spark gap which will stimulate the scalp without causing the client discomfort.

After use, clean all electrodes which have been used, remembering that if you use some type of spirit (alcohol) the electrodes must be allowed to dry for some time before using on another client.

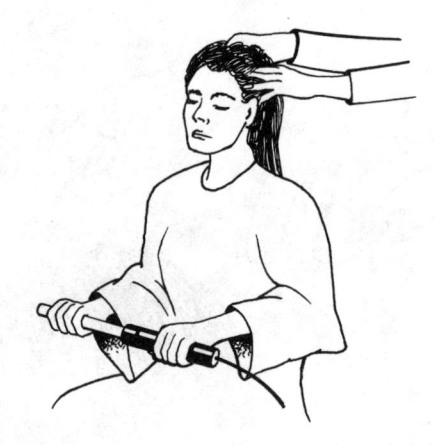

Fig. 7.10 Indirect high frequency treatment.

7.6 Questions

1. Why are treatments a potential area for growth in salon services?
2. Why might you benefit from using a major manufacturer's range of conditioning products?
3. Are there any benefits attached to selling your own range of products?
4. What is a conditioner?
5. For what reasons do we need conditioners?
6. Why is hair more damaged near its points?
7. What are the main differences between physical and chemical hair damage?
8. What types of conditioner are there?
9. Why are some conditioners substantive to hair?
10. What are the three main categories of conditioner?
11. What are oil conditioners used for?
12. Why do they give the hair lustre?
13. What were acid conditioners originally used for?
14. What effect have they on the hair and why are they useful to use after chemical processing?
15. Describe how different substantive conditioners affect the hair.
16. What is a protein hydrolysate?
17. Why are protein conditioners used on damaged hair before processing?
18. What does a hair restructurant do?

19 How would you apply a conditioner?
20 Why should all the conditioner be rinsed from the hair?
21 How can heat be applied during a conditioning treatment?
22 What is the difference between surface and penetrating conditioners?
23 Why might you perform an oil treatment?
24 Describe how you would give an oil treatment.
25 Why do you use undiluted shampoo to remove the oil?
26 What is massage?
27 What effects has massage on the scalp?
28 What are the contra-indications to massage?
29 How should you prepare yourself to give a massage?
30 Briefly describe the five basic massage techniques.
31 Which two movements would you use mostly?
32 How would you perform the friction movement?
33 What is a 'Stimulux' machine?
34 What is a vibro and what type of applicator would be used directly on the scalp?
35 When might you use high frequency?
36 What are the contra-indications for high frequency?
37 How would you carry out a high frequency treatment directly?
38 How would you carry out a high frequency treatment indirectly?

8
Specialised Hair Work

All hairdressers want to be able to satisfy their clients' needs by being able to meet each individual client's requirements. If the hairdresser is unable to carry out a particular request, it could result in the loss of a client to another salon where that service is available.

Styling long hair is often a frightening prospect for the hairdresser, but it need not be. We all remember the people who can work with long hair as if it were second nature – the ones who have a 'feel' for the hair. If you are not one of that minority, read on! In this chapter we will be looking at simple ways of achieving styles for long hair and also at adding false hair to create stunning looks on shorter hair. Once the principles of these skills are mastered, only the hairdresser's imagination will limit the originality and intricacy of the work that is produced.

8.1 Putting up hair

All hairdressers need to be able to put up long hair. It can be unsettling when you are learning this to watch someone deftly handle a mass of hair and transform it into a beautifully elegant dressing. There are some simple techniques which can be learnt and practised so that you need never fear the next time a client asks you to put up her hair.

8.2 Simple chignons

The term 'chignon' was originally used to describe a hairpiece worn at the nape of the neck to create a low roll, knot, twist or woven dressing.

Specialised Hair Work

Today, this term is also used to describe a wide range of hairstyles for longer hair that incorporate a combination of rolls, twists, pleats or knots.

Preparation of the hair for a chignon

The hair should be clean and dry. Some styles do not require the hair to be set on rollers before working; these are usually the ones which do not require backcombing. If the hair does require setting it can either be done using ordinary setting rollers or heated rollers for a quicker result. Obviously, when using rollers, the rollers should be placed in the direction of the intended style. If the hair does not require setting, shampoo and dry the hair using a blow drier. Tongs or a hot brush can be used to add any movement that is required.

Make sure that the hair is thoroughly brushed before beginning to dress the hair. Applying a little gloss cream to the hair will help reduce any static in the hair, making it more manageable as well as giving it a good sheen. Do not apply too much or the hair will become heavy and greasy.

Where you begin dressing the hair will depend upon the look you are creating. Some styles will need to be dressed in a specific area before moving onto the next one. Plan your dressing so that you do not disturb your previous work. Always try to work cleanly. Nothing looks worse than having backcombing or pins showing.

How to make a woven chignon — step by step

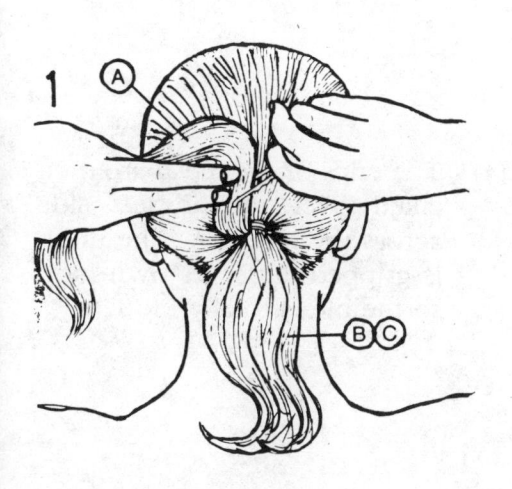

(1) Brush all the hair back off the face and secure into a ponytail at the nape of the neck. Use a covered elastic band to secure the hair; this imposes little stress on the hair and so minimises damage. Any fine, loose hairs can be held in place by spraying with hairspray and lightly smoothing them down with your hand. Divide the ponytail into three equal-sized meshes and grip the mesh A securely as shown in the diagram.

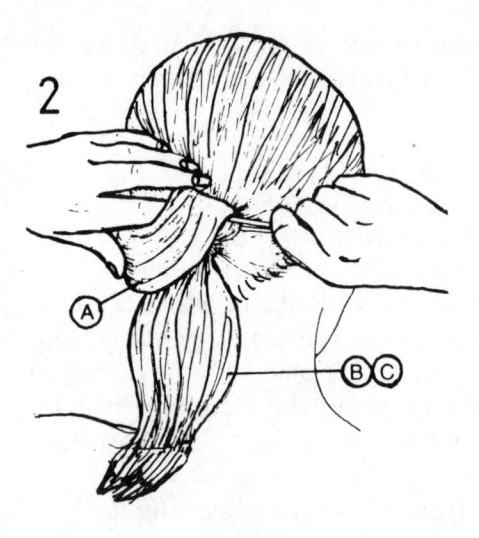

(2) Still working with A, twist it back towards the nape and grip it so that the ends of the hair are neatly tucked in.

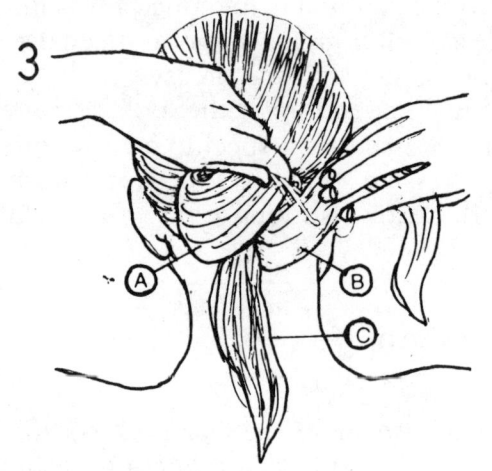

(3) Divide the loose hair into two equal meshes, B and C. The one on the right hand side in the diagram is B, and this should be directed upwards and gripped.

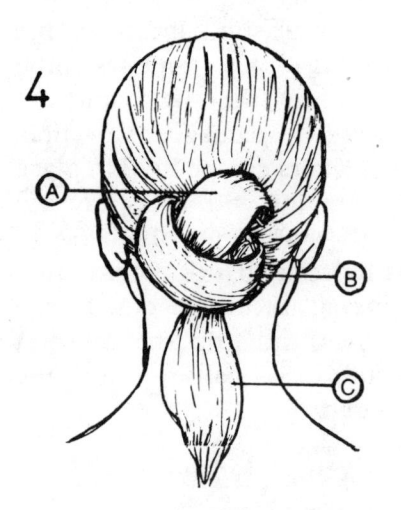

(4) The ends of the mesh are then taken over to the left side across the top of A. The mesh is gripped under its own loop so the pin is totally hidden.

Specialised Hair Work

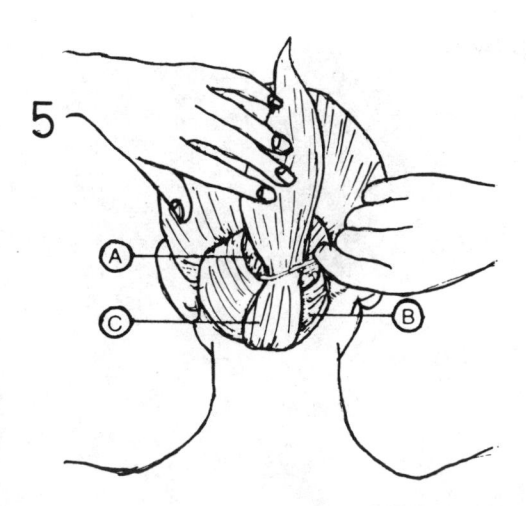

(5) The final mesh of hair, C, is taken straight up over both A and B and gripped under the first loop, A.

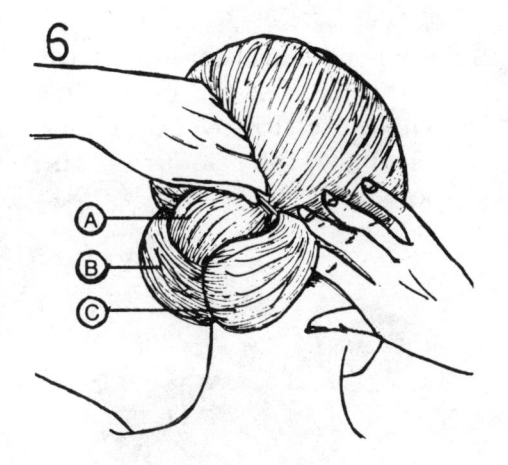

(6) The ends of C are then taken over to the right hand side and gripped into a loop so that the ends are tucked in and the pins are hidden.

196 Cutting and Styling: a salon handbook

How to make a plaited chignon — step by step

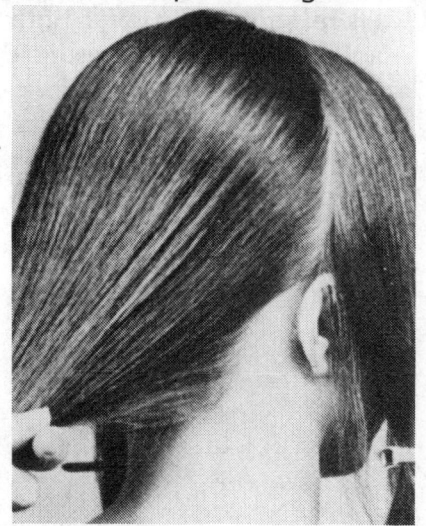

(1) Make a centre parting from forehead to crown. Make another parting across the top of the head from ear to ear. (Illustrations courtesy of Pivot Point.)

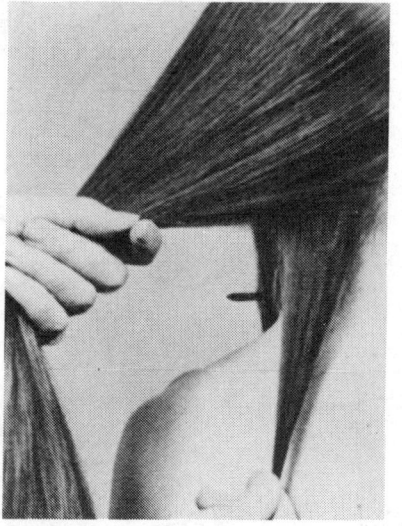

(2) Take out a small amount of hair at the nape of the neck. This will be used to cover the elastic band which secures the ponytail.

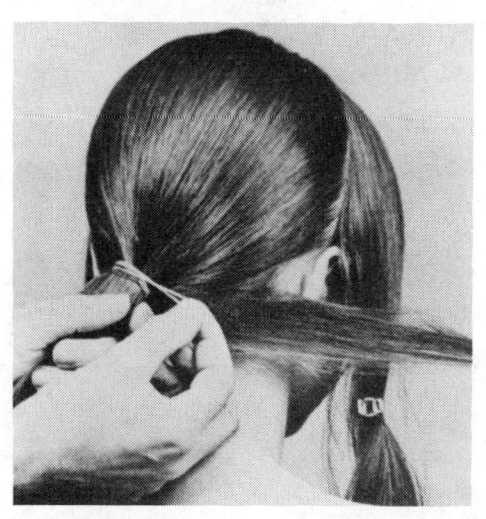

(3) Leaving out the small mesh of hair that has been purposely freed, secure the hair into a ponytail close to the head, using an elastic band.

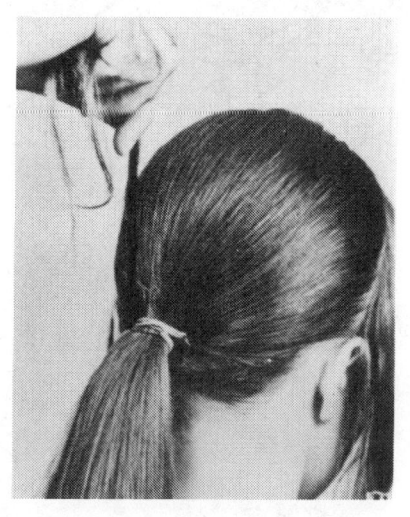

(4) Wrap the small strand around the elastic band to conceal it.

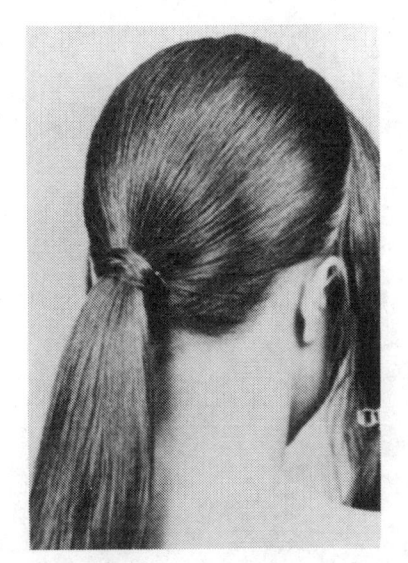

Specialised Hair Work **197**

(5) To keep this strand in place, lightly spray with hairspray and secure with a pin or grip.

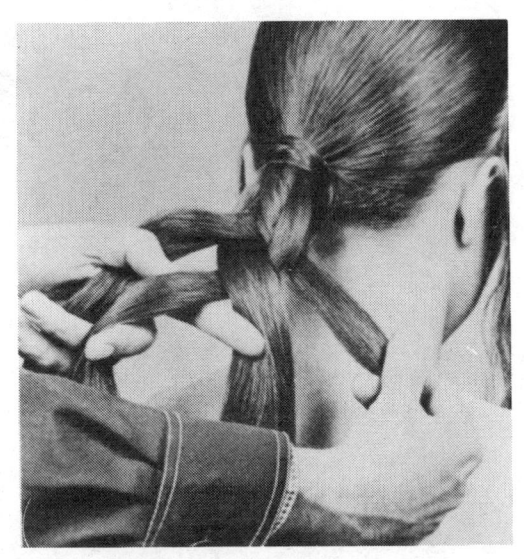

(6) Divide the ponytail into four equal strands and make a four stem plait.

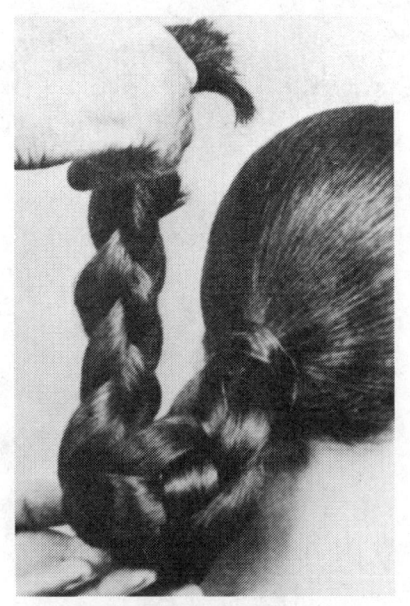

(7) When plaited, lightly backcomb the ends and spray to hold the plait. Bring the braid up, folding it on itself, taking the ends of the plait around the base of the ponytail.

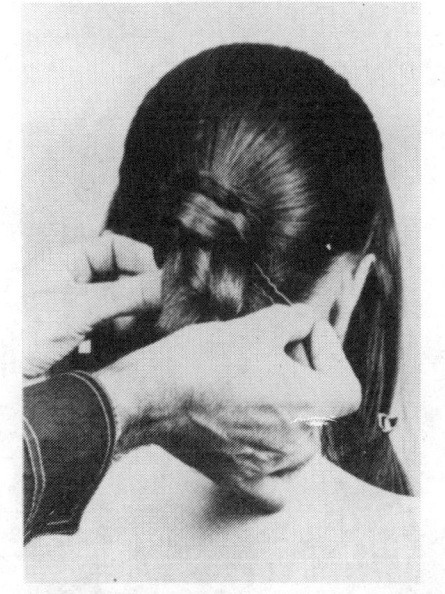

(8) Pin the plait securely using metal setting pins.

198 Cutting and Styling: a salon handbook

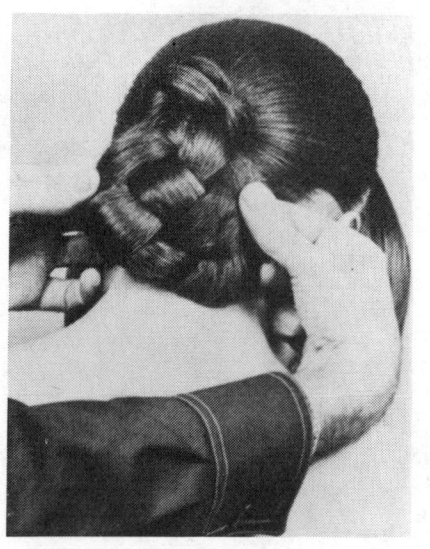

(9) Using your fingers, spread the plait to widen it.

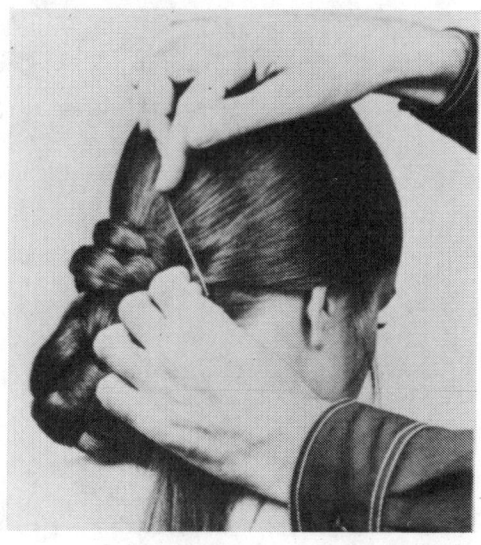

(10) Brush back the hair at the side and secure it close to the plait using grips.

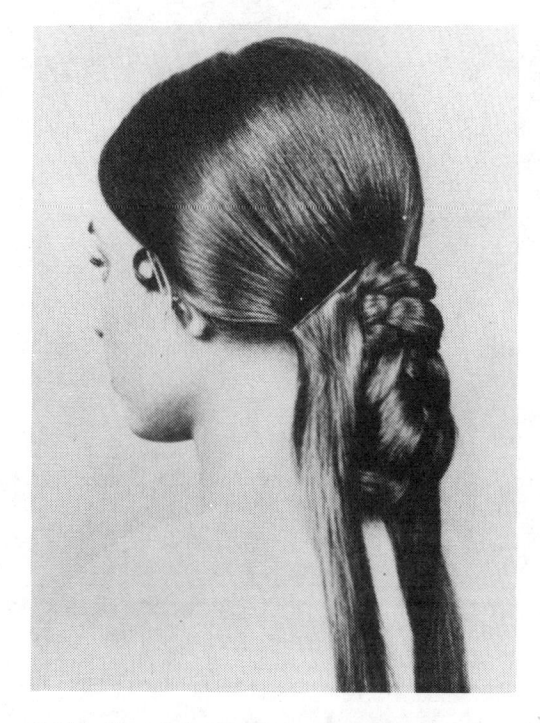

(11) Do this to the other side as in the photograph.

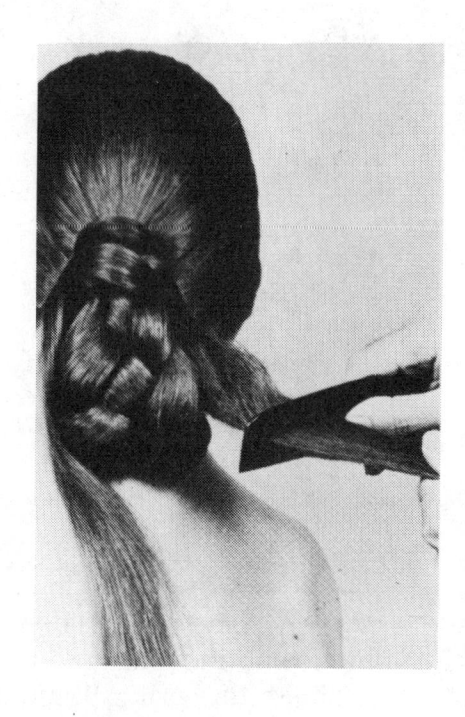

(12) Backcomb both of these strands to give them volume and width.

Specialised Hair Work 199

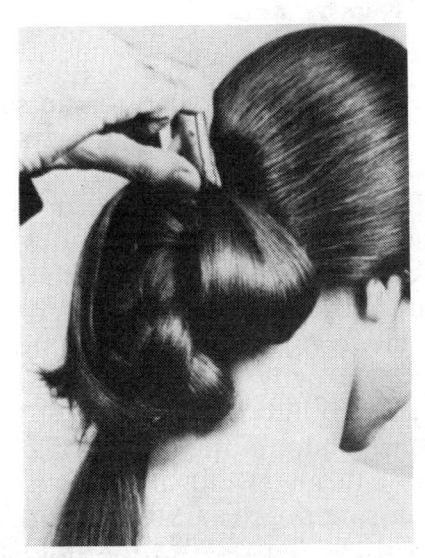

(13) Smooth the strands in an upward movement and secure them to the base of the plait. The ends of the strand are made into a small loop.

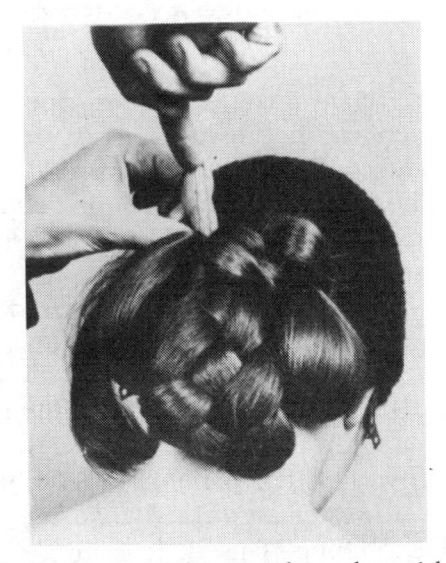

(14) Repeat this on the other side, ensuring that both are evenly balanced.

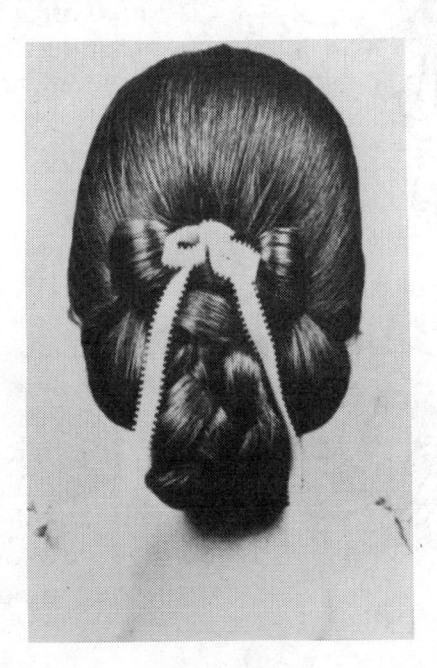

(15) The final dressing, which has been ornamented with a ribbon.

8.3 How to make a French pleat — step by step

The French pleat is perhaps one of the most versatile ways of dressing longer hair because the top hair can be styled in a variety of ways to produce a number of different looks.

The hair can either be set on ordinary or heated rollers for a French pleat or can be dressed without any preliminary preparation. This style is dressed in two distinct stages; the sides and back are styled first and then the top hair is styled. It can be dressed with or without backcombing, although some backcombing will give greater control to the hair and shape that are created, and the grips will not slip on the hair quite as much because they will have something to grip on to. From a profile view, the actual fold of hair at the back of the head which forms the pleat should be narrowest at the nape, gradually becoming fuller towards the crown, so that it creates an attractive shape, emphasising the shape of the head. If backcombing is used, it is important that it is not seen in the finished dressing, as should be true for any style.

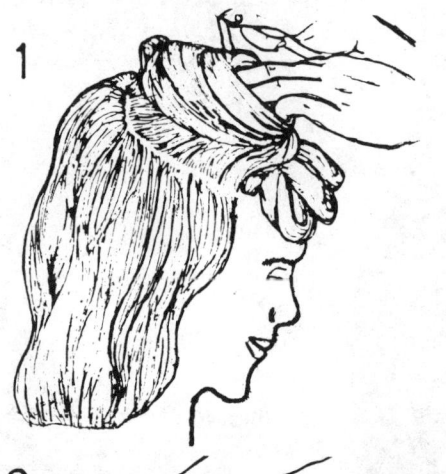

(1) Divide the hair into two main sections as shown in the diagram, so that a square-shaped section of hair is parted off at the top, front of the head, and is fastened out of the way with a clip.

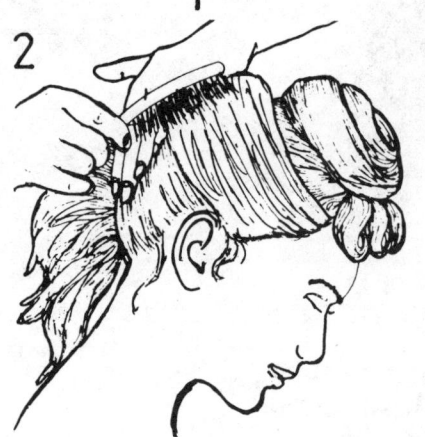

(2) If you intend to use backcombing, do this by holding the hair meshes in the direction of the intended style (i.e. directional backcombing), backcombing the meshes from underneath. Using a small bristle brush or comb, sweep the hair over to one side of the head as shown in the diagram.

Specialised Hair Work

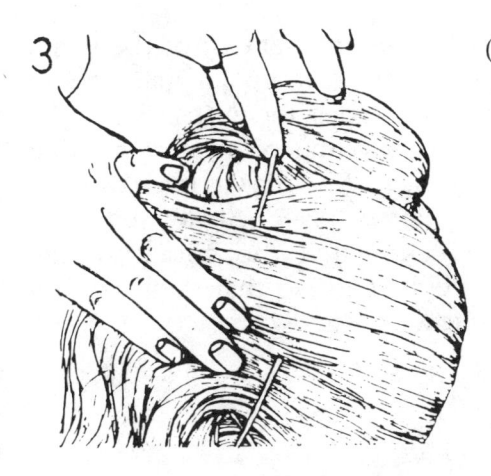

(3) To secure the hair in this position, begin placing grips on the centre back of the head, starting at the nape. The grips should cross over each other as shown at the bottom of the diagram; they will hold the hair more securely this way. Make sure the hair at the nape is directed in an upwards movement as this tends to lengthen the neck, making the back view more attractive.

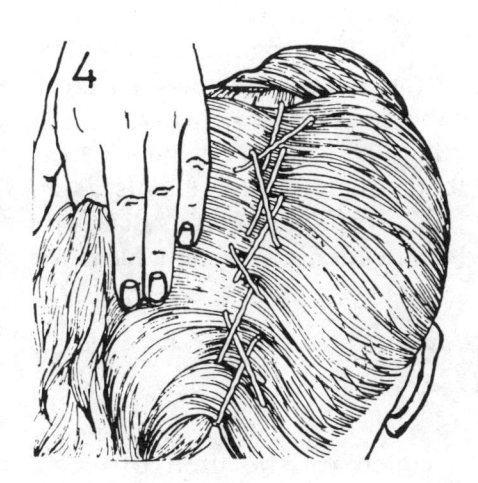

(4) Once the grips are securely in position as shown in the diagram, begin to gather the loose hair together, being careful not to disturb the pinned hair.

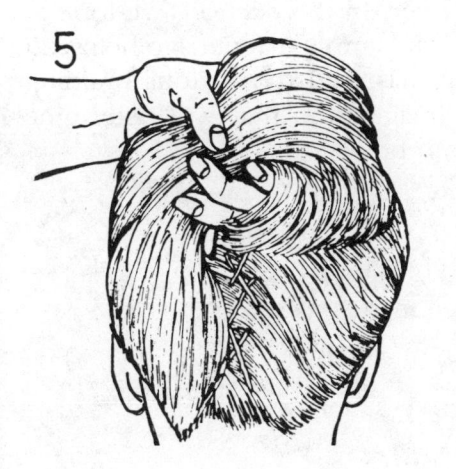

(5) The loose hair is now brought over to the middle of the head in one hand as shown in the diagram. Care should be taken so that no loose hair is left behind.

202 Cutting and Styling: a salon handbook

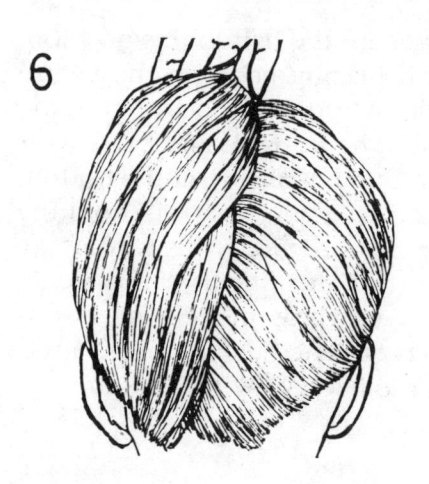

(6) With one movement of the hand, twist the hair up and around so that it hides the grips. Tuck the ends into the pleat, and without letting go, use pins to keep the fold of hair in place. Always use pins which match the colour of the client's hair, so that they will not show easily.

The top hair can now be dressed in position. The original French pleat was symmetrical and dressed fairly high, although there are many different ways to dress the top to produce fashionable looks.

It is interesting to note that the hair need not be long to be able to dress it into a French pleat, so it is a look that you can offer clients as an alternative to their current style. Exotic hair ornaments such as diamanté slides, combs and flowers, can be used to decorate a French pleat for special occasions such as weddings.

8.4 Plaiting or braiding long hair

Plaiting or braiding long hair is a skill which can be used to create interesting and stunning looks for longer hair. In this section, we look at methods of braiding hair with the use of clear, simple diagrams to help you master these techniques. Once you have mastered the various braiding techniques, it is only the limits of your imagination that will determine how intricate and original your designs can be.

Specialised Hair Work

How to make a two strand braid — step by step

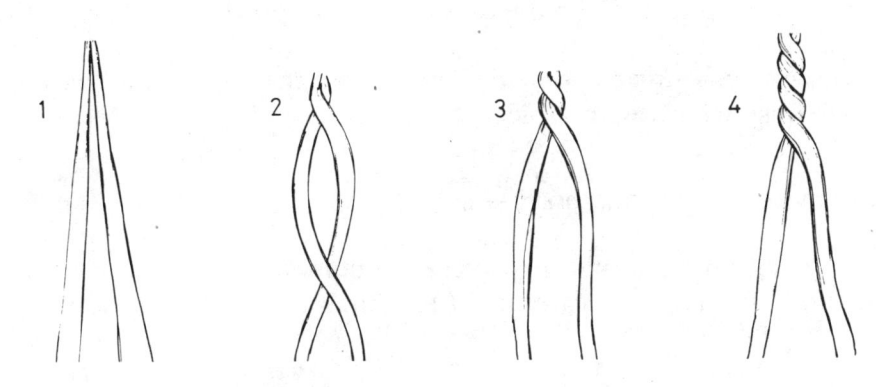

(1) Separate the section into two equal parts. (Illustrations courtesy of Pivot Point.)
(2) Cross the sections over each other.
(3) Continue crossing the hair strands over each other, being careful to maintain even tension on the strands.
(4) Cross the strands over each other along the entire length. When you reach the ends, secure with a pin, or tie with thread without letting go.

How to make a three strand braid — step by step

This is perhaps the most common of all braiding techniques.

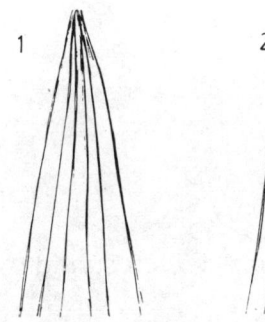

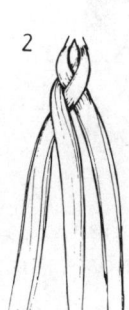

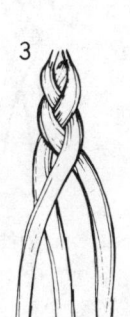

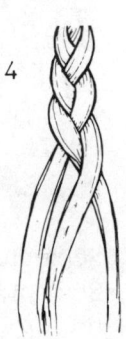

(1) Separate the section into three equal parts. (Illustrations courtesy of Pivot Point.)
(2) Begin by crossing one of the strands on the outside across the one in the centre. Then cross the other outside strand across the centre one. In the diagram, you can see that the strand on the right side is the next one to be crossed over to the centre.

204 Cutting and Styling: a salon handbook

(3) In this diagram it is the strand on the left that now needs to be crossed over to the centre. Keep the tension even to produce a regular shaped braid.

(4) Continue crossing the outside strands into the centre until you reach the ends. Secure with a piece of thread or a pin.

How to make a four strand braid — step by step

The four strand braid looks very intricate but is really quite easy to master if you study the diagrams carefully. (Illustrations courtesy of Pivot Point.)

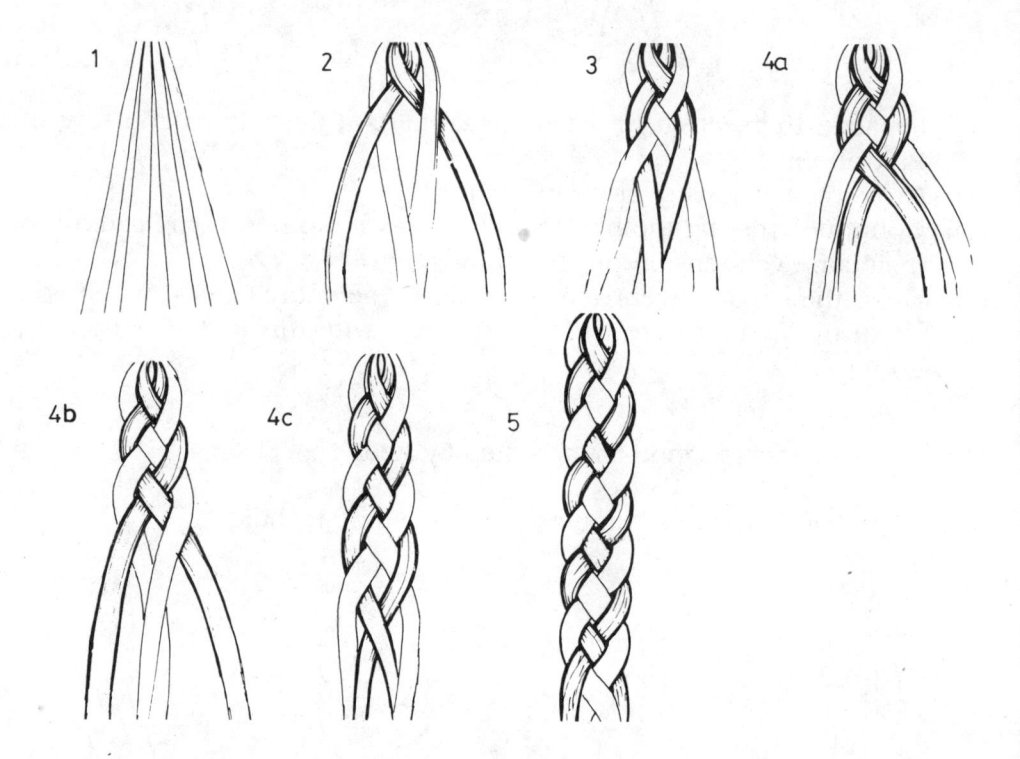

(1) Separate the section into four equal parts.
(2) Start braiding with the two centre strands, taking the left strand over the right one.
(3) The side strand is then brought to the centre by bringing the one on the right side *above* one of the first two strands, and the strand on the left side is taken *under* the other one.
(4) Diagrams 4(a), (b) and (c) show how this is continued along the hair length with the two centre strands always being crossed in the same manner as in number 2.

Specialised Hair Work

(5) The finished braid is shown in this diagram. It can be fastened by a covered elastic hair band or ribbon. A needle with a large eye can be used to weave coloured thread or ribbon through the braid to create a stunning effect for special occasions. This looks particularly effective if it has a metallic coating.

How to make an eight strand braid — step by step

This braid is more difficult to master because you will probably feel that you need an extra pair of hands! Braiding with this number of strands is much easier to do if you have somebody to help you hold and control the hair as you are working. An eight-strand braid will be shown at its best on very long hair.

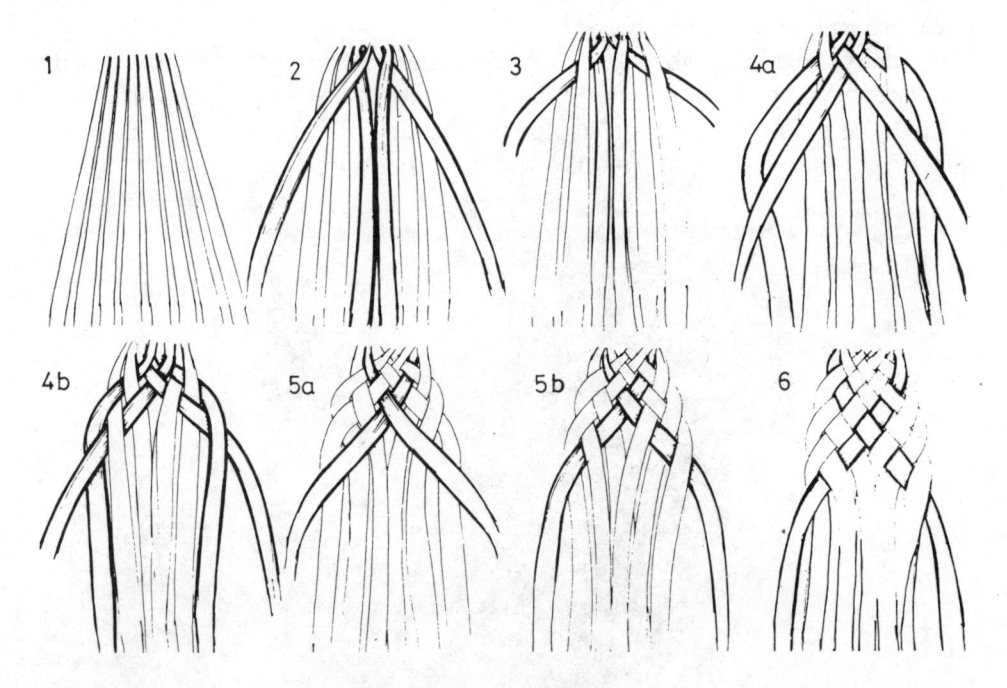

(1) Separate the section into eight equal parts.
(2) Begin by crossing the four centre strands, two by two. Take the strands on the right over those on the left (study the diagram carefully).
(3) Weave these strands out to the edges by taking them over and under the other strands.
(4) Diagrams 4(a) and (b) now take the two centre strands again and cross these left over right, as shown in 4(a) and (b).
(5) Continue weaving out towards the edges, keeping an even, slight tension to make the braid even, as shown in 5(a) and (b).

(6) Continue in this way to the hair points, securing the ends with thread or pins. Once you have mastered the eight strand braid, try a sixteen strand braid following the same pattern as you did with this one!

8.5 Hair extensions

It was Simon Forbes at the Antenna salon in Kensington, London, who pioneered the idea of adding acrylic fibre to heads of hair to create stunningly interesting looks.

Monofibre extensions come in bright colours such as pink, blue and green, or more neutral shades to blend with the wearer's natural hair colour. They can be used for creating wild looks, or used to add length and bulk to short hair which can then be cut to style for less outrageous clients. They are extremely versatile.

Basically, the false fibre is attached to the client's real hair by braiding and then heating the fibre (which melts) to form a strong seal. Some salons use a flame to do this, but on grounds of safety this should not be done, so stick to an electric apparatus like the one illustrated in Fig. 8.1.

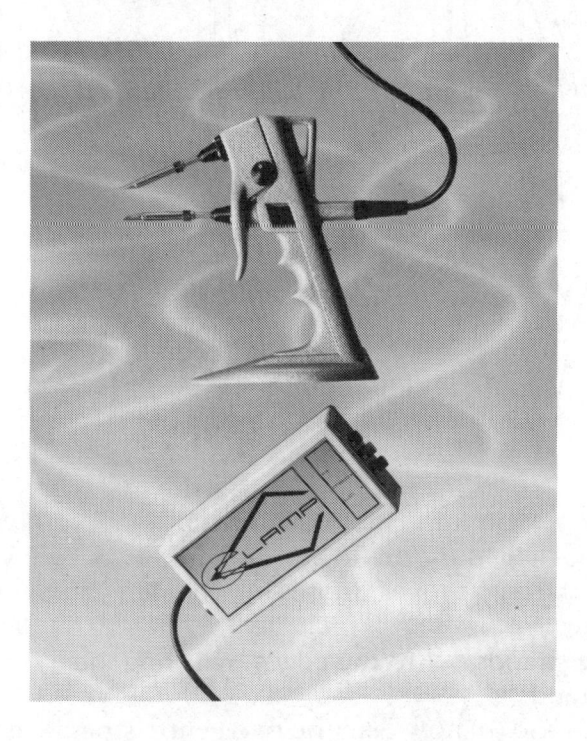

Fig. 8.1 The Clamp is an electric implement used to seal monofibre to the hair. It is thermostatically controlled and safe to use. (Courtesy of Antenna Ltd.)

Extensions can be attached in many imaginative ways. The most popular are called 'warlocks' 'ragtails', 'dreadlocks', 'cable curls', 'monofines' (see Fig. 8.2) and 'bobtails'. Each technique creates a different look which is guaranteed by Antenna to last for a minimum of three months. As their clients come from as far afield as Switzerland and Sweden, it is not unusual for the extensions to be worn in the hair for as long as a year! However, Antenna do emphasise that the extensions are harder to remove if they are left in the hair for such long periods.

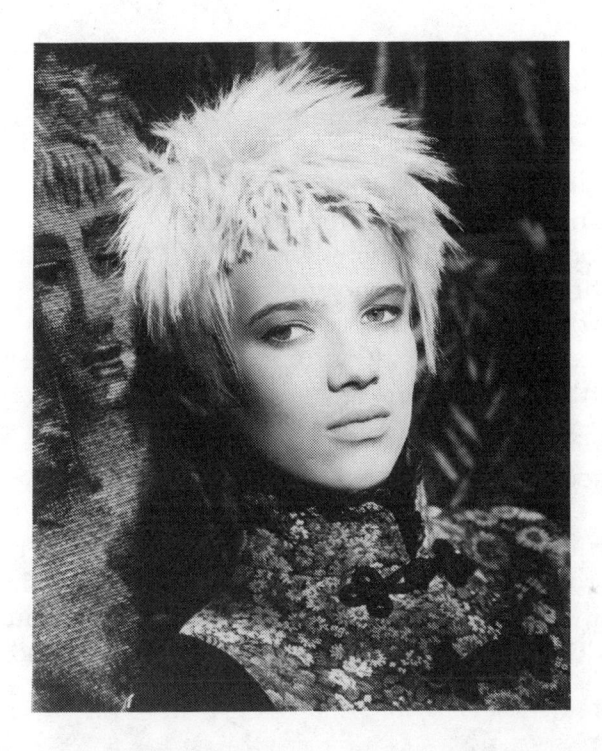

Fig. 8.2 The 'Dodger'. A soft-textured style that retains a definite shape. Monofines have been scattered through the head, then clipper-cut freehand. (Courtesy Antenna Ltd.)

How are extensions applied?

In an average situation, sixty extensions would be applied. Attaching extensions takes a long time, usually over two hours, and requires two stylists because two pairs of hands are needed. One pair of hands act as the 'control' hands, while the others use a four-stem braid to join the fibre with the client's own hair (see technical tips, below).

Once the fibre is attached to the real hair by the braiding, it must be sealed in position. As we said previously, this can be done with a naked flame, such as a candle. This chars the fibre rather than just melting it, and is also a possible fire hazard in the salon. A special piece of salon equipment called the 'Clamp' has been specifically designed for the sealing of monofibre extensions. It is illustrated in Fig. 8.1 and has the following advantages:

- It can be used to seal the finer extensions called monofines.
- It can be used to attach extensions much closer to the scalp than a naked flame.
- It reduces the operating time.
- It creates a more professional image.
- It melts rather than chars monofibre.

The Clamp is hand-cast and finished, and is made from solid aluminium. The two nickel-plated tips are heated electrically and can be detached for cleaning with something like fine emery paper. They are thermostatically controlled by three buttons on the control unit. The trigger on the Clamp controls the movement of the two heated tips. When the trigger is squeezed the tips close on the monofibre, sealing the extension in place by melting it onto the natural hair.

How are extensions removed?

Extensions take just as long to remove as they do to apply. The bond made by the heat is broken by twisting it from side to side, and the braid is then unravelled until the monofibre is separated from the natural hair. The extensions could be removed at home by the client, with the aid of a friend.

What advice should be given to the client who has extensions?

It is a good idea to design an after-care leaflet which can be taken away by the client. It should contain the following information and advice:

- Allow two weeks before shampooing and then use cool water and massage gently.
- Brushing or combing is not advisable.
- General 'bunching' normally occurs within a period of two weeks. This is considered to be part of the look and style of extensions.
- To avoid tangling at the roots, it is advisable to run the fingers gently through the roots every couple of weeks.
- Explain how the extensions can be removed at home.
- Extensions will loosen due to natural hair growth.

Technical tips

- Lift extensions at the front of the head so that you can cut them over your hands. This will prevent hitting the eyebrows or eyelashes whilst clipper cutting.
- Razor cutting can make the extensions look more real as they blend in with the natural hair better.
- Cut monofibre extensions with a separate pair of scissors which you don't value too highly. The monofibre will dull scissor blades.
- Cut up bales of monofibre using ordinary needlework scissors.
- When creating a haircut use a free-hand approach, relying on what you can see and feel.
- Encourage staff to wear extensions in different styles; they are suitable for many types of client.
- Make extensions thicker at the back of the head. Concentrate your fine extensions on the sides and front of the head.
- Advise clients that extensions tend to moult for up to 24 hours after the service. They should not fall out, so make your client aware of this in case they come back complaining – that is never good for business!
- Monofibre does not absorb tint. If ever you bleach hair with extensions scattered throughout the hair, rinse the head four of five times longer than normal after bleaching. Any bleach remaining under the extension could cause breakage.
- You might find it beneficial to take deposits on appointments for extensions if it is not a regular client. With two stylists involved it means booking out over two hours for each operator. If someone will not leave a small deposit (or even a post-dated cheque) they are unlikely to turn up for the appointment.

8.6 Questions

1. What did the term 'chignon' originally mean?
2. How should rollers be placed?
3. Briefly describe how to make a woven chignon.
4. Briefly describe how to make a plaited chignon.
5. Briefly describe how you would make a French pleat.
6. How might you decorate a French pleat for a special occasion?
7. Using coloured pencils for the different parts of the section, draw diagrams of how to make: (a) a two strand braid; (b) a three strand braid; (c) a four strand braid (d) an eight strand braid.
8. How might you use extensions in your work?

9   Why is the heated Clamp preferred to a naked flame to melt the monofibre?
10 How are extensions removed?
11 What advice would you give a client with extensions on leaving the salon?
12 What do you consider the most important technical tips when using extensions?

9
Salon Organisation

Many students who have attended colleges, whether full- or part-time, have switched off at the first mention of the words 'business studies' or 'salon organisation'. But they could find themselves amongst one salon owner in five who are forced out of business each year. If you are studying for examinations, or just interested in some of the rudiments of running a business, read on. Everyone should aspire to work for themselves one day.

9.1 Finding the ideal salon

So you have enough experience to run your own salon. You probably have set ideas about how your ideal salon should look and the type of clientele you would like to attract. The salon that you buy or rent must match these ideals.

Should I rent or buy?

This depends on how much money you have to start with, or how much you can attract. Many excellent hairdressers are 'backed' by somebody who has confidence in their ability. This can be an ideal arrangement because it can give you the chance to become established without taking a financial gamble yourself. Invest money in a solicitor to check any contracts that you might sign, in case you sign away rights like trading under your own name or your shop name. If you want to open up a shop with the minimum of capital outlay you would do best to rent. Also there may not be much choice of property to buy in many towns because most property will be leased rather than sold outright. Many shops will be 'lock up' while others will have a flat above them where you could live, or rent to someone else to provide more income. Start searching once you have some idea of the finance required; look in local property papers and trade journals. Some estate agents also lease and sell commercial properties. Don't buy a shop which has not been a hairdresser's before until you have permission from the local council to run it as a business. If you took over a clothes shop next door to an already established hairdresser's they could object, and in many cases you would not be able to open.

What about the area?

The general area that you find your ideal salon in is very important. If you want a salon that attracts young people, find an area with new housing or be in town near shops and offices. If shampoos and sets are your cup of tea, go for an older area of housing, with old people's homes or flats nearby. A men's salon would be ideal in an area with banks and offices. This will often mean early closing hours in the week and no opening on Saturdays – the City of London, for example, is like a ghost town at weekends. Go back to the area several times, at different times on different days. Check other local shops to see what type of people use them. If the local butcher sells only the cheaper cuts of meat, the people are unlikely to be big spenders on hairdressing. If you open the wrong type of salon for an area, no matter how splendid the salon is, it will almost certainly fail.

What else should I take into account about the location?

The first thing to check is how easy it is to get to? Is there more than one passing bus route and could clients park nearby? Will people know your salon is there? If it is on the first floor they will only notice an entrance doorway and will be less likely to chance a visit if they cannot see inside. Go for a ground floor salon so that you can have attractive window displays. Elderly clients might find stairs difficult. Be extremely careful of the nearby shops. You don't want to be next door to a fish and chip shop or a curry house as the smells might be off-putting. Similarly, being next door to an undertaker's would not be the best way to attract older clients. Supermarkets have their pros and cons; the people who use them generally rush in to fill their trolleys and then rush home before their frozen food melts. But they may notice you and come back. Good shops to be near include post offices, chemists or off-licences; these attract customers to an area – pensioners to cash their pensions or buy stamps, others to fill prescriptions or buy drink for parties. You will get noticed by people who might not otherwise come to a parade of shops. Check the area for other salons. Sometimes there are far too many. Opening almost next door to a busy salon is suicide, as you will look even emptier than you are, and empty salons do not inspire the confidence of the public. There may be smart shopping arcades in your town. If these are Regency or Victorian, how about opening a shop that reflects the original period in decor and staff uniforms? This has proved very successful in some towns and clients do not mind paying the more modern prices!

I've found an empty shop in a good location, what else should I think of?

First, is the building in good condition? Check for dampness in the plaster and large cracks in the walls. Has it got central heating, which is essential for the comfort of your clients but expensive to have installed. If so, is it gas, electric or oil? Remember you will be paying the running costs so find out what they are. Is there enough room, for reception, tinting and shampoo areas, for example? What would it be like if several clients were receiving attention and several more were waiting? Think ahead to when you are successful on a busy Saturday afternoon! With the public in your salon you will need to provide toilet facilities. Is there enough room for a staff-room as well as stock and a laundry area? Check with a builder how much it would cost to get everything just right for opening as a salon; he will be able to advise you on water and electricity supplies as well as drainage. You will almost certainly need new circuits for electrical equipment like drier banks, which can be expensive.

What about opening a salon in a large store?

Of course this is something that has been done on a large scale in recent years by the larger hairdressing chains. Harrods, for example, has one of the largest salons in the world within it. There are new shopping complexes being built outside large towns, and these feature many services including hairdressing. To aim for this you really need to have absolute confidence in the store, since it would be bringing in the customers you are hoping to attract. Before you sign a contract have it checked by a solicitor first, so that you can have its terms and conditions explained to you in everyday language. If the store closes every night at 5.30 pm will this suit you? Check whether you have to contribute towards the cost of contract cleaners, heating and lighting, rates, parking facilities (if any exist for you and your staff) as extras or are they inclusive in the rent. Before you commit yourself, learn all the facts about running costs. As an alternative, you may prefer the idea of opening a salon in an hotel. Many hotels like this idea and currently many very successful older-style barber shops are opening in hotels, not only in this country, but around the world.

Whom should I consult before making the final decision?

If the building is not already a salon check with the local council to see if you can change the use of premises. This is usually no problem, unless objections are raised by other traders already in the area whose trade you might affect.

If the building is already a salon you will be allowed to have the books examined by an accountant. This is important; remember that the turnover of money per week does not take account of rates, rent, electricity, gas, phones, laundry, stock, staff and salon refurbishment; a very impressive total might dwindle down to a few pounds profit eventually. An accountant will be able to forecast an average weekly profit margin as he will look at the low points and the high points of the year, as well as finding any figures 'hidden' by another accountant!

Have the fabric of the building checked if you are buying. There could be many hidden defects in a building, such as damp, dry rot, subsidence or a faulty roof. You might need thousands of pounds to put these right, so check first!

Don't visit a bank manager until you are sure of your sums. He will want to know what you want and why before he can consider offering it to you. The bank will expect you to have some money yourself.

Contact an insurance broker to find out the best prices for policies to insure yourself, your staff, the building and its contents, and your clients.

Finally, get everything checked by a solicitor before you sign anything. Try not to cut corners here as you are protecting yourself and the solicitor is often an invaluable source of information. Along with your accountant, he may direct you towards government schemes to save you money on taxes and rates while you start a new business. There are often grants for starting a business in certain areas. Money may also be provided towards wages if it is a new business, and the intricacies of the YTS scheme need to be understood before you grab a school-leaver as a junior. Remember that some kind of off-the-job training must be allowed for; YTS trainees cannot be chained to a shampoo basin for six days a week or you will have the MSC taking away your allowance!

Finally, only go ahead if you are confident about the move into business. It could mean a few years without a holiday and can put a strain on the most stable of relationships if it should go wrong.

9.2 The clients

Certain days in your life will be very exciting – your wedding day, the days your children are born, the day you pass your driving test. The day you open your own salon should be a similar event. The sad fact about this is that however exciting it is for you it will not be anything like as exciting for the general public! Don't expect them to be waiting to break down the salon door as it opens and appear in their droves if they know nothing about it. There are ways and means of letting them know, but generally these are expensive. Your advertising must therefore be financially realistic. If you buy an already existing salon there may be a certain amount of 'goodwill' sold with it. This should mean that the departing owner has not told his old clients that he is opening somewhere else or is happy to come to their homes to do their hair. Unfortunately for your business this does sometimes occur, especially if you do not keep on some of the old staff. We have known some salons where the owner has introduced his staff to their new boss last thing on a Saturday night to try to avoid this problem! Even if your shop has this goodwill (which you generally are paying for as part of the purchase price) don't rely on it. The old maxim 'it pays to advertise' has a lot of truth in it. There are several methods to advertise:

(1) television;
(2) radio;
(3) newspapers;
(4) posters;
(5) leaflets;
(6) Yellow Pages or Thompson Local Directories.

(1) Television.
So we always start off by thinking big! It is unfortunate that the very high cost of advertising a salon on television cannot possibly be paid back in the clientele it attracts. Clients are only going to come to your salon if they live or work within a certain distance of your shop, so much of this advertising could be worthless. One day there may be more cable television and then it could become a financial possibility. Otherwise you have to do something like a charity haircutting event and get one of the local programmes to cover it. Celebrity openings of salons may get local newspaper coverage but not television. If you can get yourself onto a game show you can always blurt out the name of the salon!

(2) Radio.
BBC radio stations don't take advertisements so you will only get a mention if you can get involved in a local news story such as a charity or sponsored event. If you are good enough, try to see if a local radio station is interested in having someone who is a hair expert on a phone-in show. This can provide really good publicity. If you decide to pay for adverts see what kind of deal you can strike up. An advert going out only once will not be reinforced; if you do not hear it properly the first time you might tend

to listen the second time to catch an address or phone number, or even attractive first week prices! A local station might offer cheaper rates the more times the advert is played. The time you choose to advertise is extremely important. If your advert goes out at around coffee or tea breaks you will get more people listening. The cost of an advert is not just the broadcasting fee, but also the cost of producing the advert. If it sounds too home-made it will not do your salon much good. Although much cheaper than television, radio may still be considered too expensive for the number of clients you attract from the investment.

(3) *Newspapers*

These advertisements can be divided into two main types, ones you pay for and ones that are distributed free. The ones which you pay for are going to be either national or local, and because of where you want to attract clients from you should only be interested in local newspapers. You can consider the free locals which are pushed through your door together with the ones you have to buy. Both will be getting to the local population as long as you choose the right edition of the paper, and both will require you to pay for your advertisement. You must consider several factors, however, before you make your final choice. If anyone *buys* a newspaper he or she is definitely going to read it, whereas if one is obtained through the door for nothing they might just put it straight into the dustbin. Your advert also needs to be professionally produced so that it creates the right image, the image that your salon is trying to project. Try to think of a way that people will cut out and keep your advert, perhaps using a coupon that will give a percentage discount during the first week of opening, or an offer of a free conditioning treatment. One of the best ways to advertise in a local paper is to get the advertisement disguised as an article or editorial feature, praising the services that you offer. People often take more notice of an indirect advert. Ask to speak to the features editor of your local newspaper about this.

(4) *Posters*

These are of great value if they are well placed in your local area, near railway or tube stations. They are very useful at the time you open up to make the salon name familiar. The design of a poster needs to be eye-catching as well as quickly informative. Why should someone who sees an advert be interested in going to your salon? It must promote your business as an individual service.

(5) *Leaflets*

These must be well designed and delivered to the people in your local area who are likely to use your salon. This is a major advantage of leaflets; they get to people near your shop. Include vouchers for opening offers. Make sure that the address and telephone number is prominent and stress how wonderful the salon and staff are. This is a particularly cost-effective method of getting new clients.

Salon Organisation

(6) Yellow Pages and Thompson Local Directories
For an entry fee you have your salon address and telephone number listed in these directories which are distributed free to the public. They are not particularly useful for a new salon, but many people find them helpful.

How do I check the effectiveness of my publicity?

This must be done at the reception desk, monitoring each new client to see where they first heard of the salon. Use symbols in the appointments book for leaflets, newspapers, etc. After a month or so, you will be able to work out what was the most effective advertising medium.

Are there other ways that I can promote my salon?

Yes. One of the most effective ways is to give the client something which they will take away with them, featuring the salon name and telephone number. Particularly effective are useful articles like handbag mirrors, matches for smokers, calender cards for wallets or purses, pens or pencils and carrier bags. Everything that leaves the salon can be placed in a carrier bag which advertises your salon to anyone who sees it in the local high street. Try to get involved co-operatively with other local businesses for things like weddings; hairdressing can be arranged as part of the service by shops that provide bridal wear, flowers or hire cars. If a local shop puts on a fashion show, offer to do the hair of the models. If people like the hair they see they will take note of your name in the programme for the future. Do promotions on products, at sale times especially, when people generally have less money because of the amount they have spent in stores.

I've got the clients, but how do I keep them?

Whatever happens, always give the client the best service possible. Advise them about their hair condition and always show that you appreciate their custom. Surprisingly few salons do this! Most salons provide refreshments and magazines. Try to make your clients feel welcome, call them by their first name if they like it and always ask them when they would like their next appointment as they leave. The client can take their business elsewhere at any time. If they are ever unhappy with your service, try to make amends immediately. Offer a free conditioning treatment or a sample shampoo to take home. If you know a regular client is ill, send her a get well card. If clients send the salon postcards from their holidays, pin them up in reception. If clients ever ask for a service that you do not provide, try to provide it before they find someone else who does.

Make your reception comfortable and inviting. Welcome clients by name and apologise for any delays. Take their coats and help them on with their gowns. Give the occasional free gift such as a key ring promoting your salon. What makes the difference between you and another nearby salon is the level of service that you offer, how much a client feels involved with you and your salon.

9.3 Being an employer

For the first time people are now working for you rather than the other way round. It can be a daunting task. You will have to recruit staff and then encounter all the problems of being an employer. As this is not a book on salon management, we have not dealt with the practicalities of bookkeeping, taxation and insurance contributions. It is worth employing a good accountant for these anyway, especially when you first start a business.

How do I find the right staff?

The first thing to decide is how many people you need to employ and exactly what you will be employing them for. If it is someone for shampooing and neutralising a junior will be adequate, whereas a stylist will be required if it is because of the increased volume of trade. If the increase in trade is purely seasonal or on particular days, get a temporary or part-timer. Once you have decided what you need, you must decide on how to find them. You can advertise in local papers or trade journals for full-time staff or ask at the local college for a past student or one who is just leaving. If it is a part-timer you might place a card in the shop window or again ask the local college. If someone can be recommended you are in the position of not having to worry about their suitability as much as someone who walks in in response to an advertisement. References cannot be relied on unless you have some knowledge of the referee or their company. Give a practical test in the salon and ask to see any certificates. Many people claim they have certain certificates without ever having to produce the evidence. Be careful when advertising not to be seen to be prejudiced against someone because of sex, colour or age. If you want younger staff, try using the word 'modern' in an advertisement as this should discourage older people. If your advertisement attracts a large response you may find it necessary to do some weeding out based on qualifications, age and experience. If you have several candidates who seem reasonable, see them all, preferably testing their skills in the salon before making a decision. Be sure that they will fit in with the salon atmosphere that you already have or you may find the rest of the staff wanting to leave, as well as having unhappy clients! Anyone who works for you should be reflecting your image of the salon.

Once you are satisfied as to abilities and personality discuss a job description and contract. This should entail the duties that you envisage for the post as well as hours, wages, period of notice, holiday and sickness pay. Consult your solicitor about such contracts. Many have a radius clause which means that an employee cannot leave the salon and work within a certain distance within the next year. This protects you from having your clients poached when someone leaves. Include a period of notice in a contract; it is often better to pay employees off than have them enticing your clients away in their remaining weeks at work.

What wages should I pay?

This is never an easy question. You cannot afford to be too generous yet you must match minimum wages as laid down by the Hairdressing Wages Undertakings Council. A minimum amount is laid down for various grades which you are compelled by law to pay your staff. Prosecution and fines can result if you ignore these minimum levels. Also check with other salon owners you know in an area. It is not unknown for salon owners to check with each other before fixing wages! You may be able to offer minimum wages with bonuses built in if a certain amount of business is done each week. This way you protect yourself from a big loss on wages as you need only pay higher rates when, and if, necessary. This also encourages staff, as they tend to think of their wages as what they could earn in a good week.

We know of many salons who pay the same basic wage whether the employee works for forty or eighty hours, but this is wrong. After forty hours (or whatever you have agreed with your staff as the normal working week) have been worked a rate of overtime should be paid. This should be time and one quarter on the employee's day off or for extra time in the evening, time and one half for extra time on a Saturday, and double time on a Sunday or public holiday. You can come to private arrangements about days off in lieu if holidays are worked.

The regulations concerning wages are enforced by the Wages Inspector, who has the power to check your records (which you had better keep!).

How should I pay my employees?

Your employees must first be given written particulars of employment (a contract of employment), within their first thirteen weeks of employment.

Specify the date of starting work in case of any future dispute. The particulars should include:

- job title and duties;
- rate of pay (either hourly, weekly or monthly);
- the number of hours in a normal working week;
- rules on sickness absence and sick pay;
- entitlement to holidays (including rate of pay for such);
- details of pension schemes;
- length of notice required (by you and them).

Employees can be paid in cash or by cheque. Your contract with them should have specified the frequency of payments, whether it be daily for part-timers, or weekly or monthly for full-timers. Each time you pay them you must provide an itemised statement of pay. This should tell them the following:

- gross wage;
- net wage;
- deductions such as National Insurance, superannuation and income tax;
- any bonus, commission or holiday pay.

Training

Keep your staff informed about modern trends in the industry and send them on commercial courses whenever possible. Enter competitions and take the trade journals. Send juniors to the local college to learn skills and take examinations that you would not be able to offer them in the salon. Attend trade shows and keep reminding staff about their attitude to their bread and butter, the clients. Once high standards are reached, it is easier to go down than up.

What rights have your employees?

Once they have worked for you for a certain amount of time their rights improve (none of these rights apply to anyone who is self-employed). If you have part-time staff who have worked eight hours or more per week for five years continuously, they will also have employment rights.

Maternity pay is payable if someone has worked for you for two years, and she will also be entitled to get her job back after the birth. She must be in your employment up to the eleventh week before the expected date of confinement and must also tell you that she wishes to return to work after the child is born. Your employee can return to work up to twenty-nine weeks after confinement. You must wait for forty-nine days to elapse after the birth of the child, then you can ask if she intends returning to work; she must reply within fourteen days or lose her right of employment with you. With a small business, if you have taken someone on in the meantime and cannot take back your former employee because of lack of work, your employee would lose her rights.

If you wish to terminate an employee's contract you must give one week's notice if they have been with you for less than two years; one week's notice for each year if below twelve years, and twelve weeks notice if above twelve years. Your employee must give you a minimum of one week's notice unless you specify a longer period in your contract with them. If the employee has been with you for more than six months you must give written reasons for dismissal. An employee can seek these within three months of the date of termination and if you do not give them within two weeks an industrial tribunal will award your former employee two weeks' wages.

If you want to get rid of employees you cannot make their life a misery; this would be known as constructive dismissal. Constructive dismissal includes suspension without pay, cutting wages, changing conditions of work or status. Your employees are protected against unfair dismissal if they have worked for you for more than one year (twenty people or more in the company) or two years (fewer than twenty people in the company). In most cases, then, we are talking about protection after two years of employment.

If your employee is protected, you must have a good reason to sack him or her. Tribunals generally have five reasons for two categories, one is fair reason and the other is fair procedure. As the name implies, if you have a fair enough reason, you will be able to dismiss an employee. These are:

- The employee is incapable of doing his or her work or is unqualified to do so (this could be on grounds of ill health).
- The conduct of the employee is so bad or inappropriate or having such an effect on other employees that his or her work cannot be done properly.
- The employee's job no longer exists, perhaps because of lack of trade, so the employee has become redundant.
- The employee cannot do his or her job without breaking the law (this one is very unlikely).
- Some other substantial reason (this could be conflict with other employees or clients, bad time-keeping, salon reorganisation, theft of products or client property, etc.

The way in which you dismiss the employee is also important, and there are five guidelines on fair procedure:

- Employees should be given at least one warning before being dismissed and given the opportunity to explain their side of the story.
- You should consider all the facts; for example, bad weather might make it unfair to dismiss because of a few days' bad time-keeping.
- You should only rely on facts that were known to you at the time. Don't find reasons afterwards.
- You do not have to prove your reason, you merely have to believe it to have been correct and to have acted like any other reasonable employer under the circumstances to protect your business.
- A tribunal will only step in if it thinks that you, as the employer, were unreasonable.

When is an employee entitled to redundancy payments?

Employees are entitled to redundancy payments if dismissed because their job is no longer necessary or because your business closes, and if they have worked for you for more than two years continuously (this does not mean that you can keep sacking and rehiring them!). If your salon has ten or more employees you must inform the Secretary of State for Employment (in practice, the local Job Centre) at least thirty days before the first dismissal occurs. You can claim a hefty percentage (around 40 per cent) of such payments from the local Redundancy Payments office by filling in the appropriate forms.

9.4 Your public responsibilities

There are numerous laws that will apply to you once you have opened your own business and are dealing with the public. Most of these are concerned with the service that you provide and the health and safety of the client.

Price lists and contracts

Your price list should be prominently displayed and should show all the charges that your client will incur. If a client asks you to tint her hair and you agree, you have made a contract to carry out that service at the price displayed. You cannot then decide that her hair needed a conditioner which she never agreed to pay for. This is why the initial consultation is so important as it avoids any bad feelings resulting from misunderstandings.

What is negligence?

You can be said to be negligent if the service that you or your staff provide goes wrong because of a lack of care on your part or theirs. This could include using products wrongly or not taking proper precautionary tests. If you or your staff burn a client's skin you are definitely negligent and deserve to pay some form of compensation. In such cases you could be taken to court. Similarly, you would be legally liable in the case of a skin reaction to a tint if the label stipulated that a skin test should have been carried out. If a perm does not take or a colour comes out wrong, simply rectify the mistake at your own expense without having to be asked, unless you are deliberately trying to ruin your business. You should always follow manufacturers' instructions as products have been designed to be used in particular ways. Remember: you are responsible for your staff.

When can I open my salon?

This is governed by the Shops Act of 1950 and 1965, although there are frequent attempts to permit Sunday trading. Generally, check with the local council who have the right to vary the rules in your area. Shops should not close later than 8 pm except for one night per week when they may stay open until 9 pm. According to these Acts you should also have an early closing day once a week, but we know many salons that don't. Sunday is still the day that the salon must close. Home hairdressers are, however, free to work what hours they choose.

The Health and Safety at Work Act 1974

This Act applies to everyone at work, including employers and employees. You must ensure the maintenance of your equipment and not allow it to be used if you know it to be damaged. Your staff must only do work that they have been properly trained to do. If you employ more than five people you must provide a written statement of general policy for health and safety, and make positive arrangements to carry it out. It should be displayed in the staff room. There should be safe means of access and exit to your salon. Any dangers that arise in the salon are up to you to correct.

Your employees are equally responsible and must not endanger their fellow employees or clients. They should not make repairs on electrical equipment, for example, if they do not know what they are doing. The regulations relating to first aid were given in Chapter 1. Remember to keep an accident book to write down even a trivial accident in case there are complications, later.

The Fire Precaution Act 1971 (amended 1976)

This act is concerned mostly with fire prevention and the provision of fire escapes. You will require a fire certificate if you employ more than twenty people at one time, having ten or more people working anywhere except the ground floor (basement, first floor, etc.) or if the building your salon is in has more than twenty people, including the rule of ten or more anywhere except the ground floor. Unless you are a small salon on the ground floor you will need to obtain a certificate from your local Fire Authority. You should have equipment to fight fires and have exits clearly marked. A fire alarm should be installed and tested every three months.

The Offices, Shops and Railway Premises Act 1963

This Act has been largely replaced by the Health and Safety at Work Act 1974, but some of it is still relevant to salons. It deals with the general cleanliness of the salon. It should be kept clean and the floors, passages and stairways must be kept free of obstructions and slippery substances. They should also be lit. Stairs must be provided with a handrail. It also stipulates minimum and maximum working temperatures; the salon should reach a temperature of 16°C within an hour of opening. All washing and toilet facilities should be kept clean and lit. If there are more than five people of mixed sexes employed, you must provide a toilet and basin for each sex. If you employ more than ten people regularly, you should really provide another toilet for the general public. Facilities for hanging up outside clothing, for eating food and drinking, must be supplied for employees. A seat should be available for every three employees. To prevent overcrowding the Act states that each employee should have forty square feet of floor space, a regulation which many salons must break on a busy Saturday. A copy of the Act should be available to staff.

Insurance

Before opening a salon you should be adequately insured and are required by law to carry public liability insurance. This will cover the cost of any claim by clients and it is available through trade organisations if you are a member. If you are not a member, either join or see an insurance broker who will fix you up with a good price. You should also insure for claims from employees and damage to the premises. Think of expensive items like plate glass windows or equipment and stock. What happens if you have to cease trading in the event of damage to the salon? Be adequately insured.

Salon Organisation   225

9.5 Career patterns

For completeness, we have included a brief section on career patterns. There are several ways in which hairdressing can be learnt as a trade. The method of institution is often picked by personal preference, financial position, age and expectations. We cannot say which is the best method, for that all depends on the individual. Whatever happens, however, you can only really get out what you put in.

Salon training

Many salons offer what is known as an apprenticeship though this is now being replaced by YTS. Apprenticeships are usually only open to young people, and someone in their twenties would find it very difficult to be taken on. In an apprenticeship, a contract was signed to bind both sides to a three year agreement. This time period seems to be changing towards two years. If either party broke the agreement, the damaged party could claim compensation. If you should enter into such an agreement as an employer or employee, it is wise to have a three month trial to see if you suit each other. Contracts can be backdated to account for the three month trial period. During the salon training most salons allow the trainee to attend a local college for one day a week to receive further practical and theoretical training. This day-release lasts two years and should lead to the City and Guilds examination in hairdressing. The salon may provide model nights for trainees to perfect hairdressing skills.

Youth Training Schemes

The YTS, as it has become known, is a training programme for school-leavers set up by the Manpower Services Commission (MSC) which is part of the Department of Employment. It is a two year training scheme which involves an element of off-the-job training. The scheme can be college- or salon-based, depending on who is acting as the managing agent. Whoever they are, they should be meeting certain criteria laid down by the MSC. This has set a national level of competence which should be met by the trainees.

College students

There are many colleges around the country that run full-time courses to train hairdressers, usually of two years' duration. These courses provide a background knowledge of science, business skills, and various subjects concerned with the industry such as men's hairdressing, manicure and make-up. You will have to be selected by interview and may require certain minimum examination passes. The course will usually lead to several nationally recognised examinations. The advantage of a college training is the broad base of knowledge you will acquire; the disadvantage is that your work will be slow when you enter the industry proper. If you are older and unemployed, some colleges now run intensive courses.

Commercial schools

There are many private schools which will try and train you in about nine months for a fee. You must have this money plus enough to live on but these schools give a really intensive practical training. You will usually get a diploma from the school, which is not nationally recognised. Many schools run excellent short courses to update skills.

Manufacturers' schools

Once you have been in the industry you will be able to attend short courses on colouring and perming at the centres run by the major manufacturers to promote their products. Other courses offered include management and fashion work.

Where can you work as a hairdresser?

Apart from salons all over the world, there are several other areas where you might work:

- health and fitness clubs;
- cruise liners;
- leisure centres;
- hospitals and residential homes;
- theatre, TV and movies;
- make-up studios;
- model agencies and photographic studios;
- mobile hairdressers;
- demonstrating and teaching in colleges or schools.

Competition work

Some hairdressers enjoy the challenge of competing in hairdressing competitions as well as working in a salon. If you win a really large competition it can make your name and possible fortune. It makes wonderful publicity for the salon you work in to have a plaque or trophy that you have won on display. Local papers will fall over themselves to write up your story. Go along and see a competition before you enter one for the first time. You will need a model who is as prepared as you to give up their time.

Whatever you do in the future, or wherever you go, enjoy your work. Once the fun is gone, work becomes a chore and it is time to change.

9.6 Questions

1. What factors should you take into account when deciding whether to rent or buy a salon?
2. What advantages would a flat above a shop give you?
3. If the shop had not been a salon before, what would you do?
4. How can the area help you to attract the right clientele?
5. What other factors would you take into account about location?
6. How would the building influence your choice of salon?
7. What factors should be considered when thinking of opening a salon in a large store?
8. Whom should you consult before making the final decision?
9. Discuss the ways in which you might try to attract clients.
10. How could you check that these were cost-effective?
11. What type of newspaper would you advertise in?
12. Give your reasons for the type of advertisement you would place?
13. What other ways could you promote your salon?
14. How would you keep your clients?
15. If you have your own salon, why should you consult an accountant?
16. How would you recruit staff?
17. What wages would you pay your staff?
18. How might you encourage them to work harder?
19. How would you pay your employees?
20. How would you keep your salon up-to-date?
21. What rights do your employees have?
22. How would you dismiss an employee?
23. When would they be entitled to redundancy payments?
24. Why should you consult with your client before a service?
25. Why should the price list be clearly displayed?
26. What is negligence?
27. How would you stop it happening?

28 How would you protect yourself against financial loss due to negligence?
29 During what hours can your salon be open?
30 What are the main facts of the Health and Safety at Work Act?
31 When would the Fire Precautions Act affect you?
32 How does the Offices, Shops and Railways Premises Act affect the salon?
33 What things should you insure against?
34 In what ways could you train to be a hairdresser?
35 What career opportunities are open to you as a hairdresser?

Glossary

accelerator: a device that produces infra-red radiation as a source of heat to speed up the chemical processing of hair.
acetic acid: the weak organic acid found in vinegar and used in acid rinses.
acid rinse: a rinse containing a weak organic acid used to close the cuticle and to neutralise alkalinity.
acids: a chemical compound that contains hydrogen ions, having a pH of below 7.0. Acids close the cuticle layer of the hair.
Afro: the term used to describe super-curly black hair.
alkaline: describes chemicals with a pH of more than 7.0, which contain hydroxide ions and open the cuticle of the hair.
allergy: a reaction to contact with something, usually seen as a change in the skin. Not everyone has an allergy, but a skin test is recommended before use for some hairdressing products to avoid allergic reactions.
alopecia: the medical term for baldness.
alpha-keratin: hair in its unstretched state.
amino acids: the small molecules that proteins are made of; in the cortex they help maintain moisture balance.
analysis: the examination of the client and his or her hair before any hairdressing procedure is carried out. It enables the client to express their desires and the hairdresser to carry them out without unnecessary damage to the hair.
anti-clockwise: an expression used to describe curl formation in a direction opposite to that travelled by the hands of a clock.
anti-oxidant rinse: a rinse containing an acid which is also a reducing agent, such as ascorbic acid, which reduces oxidation damage in hair.
applicators: the attachments which can be fitted to a vibro machine.

arrector pili: the muscle attached to the hair follicle which, on contraction, causes the hair to stand on end.
asymmetrical: not evenly balanced.

backbrushing: brushing back from points to roots to add volume to the hair, hairs becoming entangled because the cuticle is damaged.
backcombing: a method of achieving support and fullness, the shorter hairs being pushed down towards the roots.
backwash: a basin in which the client is washed by placing the back of the neck into the basin. It is much safer when using strong chemicals.
baldness: lack of hair in a place where it would be considered normal to have hair.
barrel curl: an open centred pincurl.
base: a mesh of hair equivalent in depth to the diameter of the roller being used and as wide as the length of the roller.
beta-keratin: keratin in its stretched condition.
blunt cut: alternative name for club cutting.
bottle trap: a trap often fitted underneath shampoo basins which prevents smells and airborne infections entering the salon. It is also easy to open if the sink becomes blocked.
braid: plaiting of hair.
bristle: animal hairs used in brushes.
buckled end: distorted points of hair caused by incorrect winding.

cape: a wrap-around protective garment used to protect the clothes of your client.
caustic: a strong alkali capable of attacking and damaging other substances. Sodium hydroxide (caustic soda), used in relaxers and to clean drains, is caustic and can damage the hair and skin.
chignon: type of long hair dressing.
citric acid: an organic acid found in citrus fruits, used in acidic rinses to neutralise alkalinity and close the cuticle of the hair.
clip: a clamp-like device used to secure the hair.
clockwise: in hairdressing, the movement of hair in the same direction as the hands of a clock.
club cutting: cutting the hair straight across to achieve blunt cut ends.
coarse hair: a hair fibre with a large diameter.
comb: an instrument used to part, dress and arrange the hair.
comb-out: the use of a hair brush or comb to open out hair into the finished style.
concentrated: condensed, usually by the removal of water; increasing the strength of a chemical solution by decreasing the bulk.
conditioner: any product applied to the hair to improve its condition.

conditioning: the application of special chemicals to the hair to help restore its strength and body.
cortex: the central layer of the hair, consisting of bundles of fibres. The natural pigment of the hair is found here.
counterclockwise: the movement of hair in the opposite direction to the hands of a clock.
cowlick: strong area of hair growth in the opposite or an unusual direction at the front hairline.
cranium: the bones of the skull which protect the brain.
crest: the raised part of a wave.
crown: the top part of the head from where the hair takes its direction of growth.
cuticle: the outer layer of the hair, consisting of several layers of overlapping scales.

damaged hair: hair which is either porous, brittle, split, dry, or has little elasticity.
dandruff: overproduction of skin scales, which are seen on the scalp. Also called pityriasis.
dense: thick, heavy.
dermatitis: inflammation of the skin as the result of being in contact with some external agent, such as perm lotion.
detergent: an agent that cleanses, a synthetic soap.
disentangle: method of removing tangles and combing the hair smooth, usually carried out with a wide-toothed comb.
dry hair: hair that lacks natural oils (sebum).

effleurage: a stroking massage movement.
elasticity: the ability of a hair to be stretched and return to its original length.
electrode: attachment for high frequency machine.
end papers: papers used to prevent buckled ends of hair.
ends: the last few centimetres (one inch) of hair, furthest away from the scalp.
epidermis: the very top layer of the skin, protecting the body from physical damage and water loss.
European hair: human hair found in Europe. For the purpose of this book reference is made to straight Caucasian hair.
evaporation: when a liquid turns into a gas.

feathering: alternative name for taper cutting.
filler: a chemical preparation that tends to equalise porosity by filling in the more porous areas.
fine hair: a hair fibre that is relatively small in diameter.

finger wave: the process of setting the hair in a pattern of waves through the use of fingers, comb and waving lotion.
follicle: the pit in the skin from which a hair grows.
French pleat: a hairstyle which is dressed so that the back hair is made into a fold.
frizz: hair having too much curl.

gel: a thick oil-in-water emulsion used to style hair.
graduation: a method of cutting which blends longer meshes of hair to a shorter perimeter shape.
guide line: the first cutting line which is made and followed throughout the entire haircut.

hairline: the edge of the scalp where the hair begins.
hair shaft: the part of the hair that projects from the skin.
hair spray: a spray used on dry hair to keep the hair in position.
hard water: water that contains calcium and magnesium salts, which will not easily form a lather with soap.
henna: a natural hair dye that can coat the hair and join with sulphur bonds in the cortex, so much so that perming may be affected.
high frequency: an alternating current used to stimulate the scalp.
hydrogen peroxide: an oxidising agent used in hairdressing, found in many neutralisers, bleaches and mixed with tints.
hydrophilic: something which is water-loving (i.e. attracted to water).
hydrophobic: something which is water-hating (i.e. repelled by water).
hygroscopic: ability of a substance (such as hair) to absorb moisture from the atmosphere.

imbrications of hair: the point where cuticle scales overlap.
infectious: something that can be caught, or passed from one client to the next.
inflammation: the reaction of the body to irritation, usually seen as an area of redness.
infra-red: a type of radiation, which is invisible and gives off heat.

keratin: the protein from which hair, skin and nails are made.
kinky: very curly hair.

lanolin: purified sheep's sebum.
lanugo: the hair found on a foetus.

Mad Mats: bendable, flat, cloth-covered templates which can be used in a variety of ways in fashion setting.

Marcel waving: a technique of forming waves in the hair by means of heated irons.
massage: manipulation of the scalp or body by rubbing, kneading, stroking or tapping, to increase circulation.
medulla: the air space found in the centre of most hairs.
melanin: the black or brown pigment found in both hair and skin.
melanocyte: the cells which produce the pigment melanin, found in the germinating layer of the epidermis.
mesh: a mesh is formed when the section is divided up, it is usually the width of the main section.
Molton Browners: flexible foam or cloth-covered rods used for setting hair.
mousse: an aerosol foam hair styling product.

nape: the name used to describe the lower part of the head.
neutral: having neither an acid nor an alkaline pH.
neutralisation: the correct chemical definition refers to the reaction between an acid and an alkali to give a salt and water and a neutral pH.

occipital: the name of the bone which forms the back of the head.
off-base: the placing of a roller so that it sits on the skin, i.e. on any hairline.
on-base: the placing of a roller so that it sits exactly on its own base, creating normal volume.
over-directed: the placing of a roller on a base which is equivalent to twice the diameter of the roller and the same length as the roller, so that it sits on the upper part of the base. This produces maximum volume.

papilla: the source of hair growth, found at the base of the hair follicle.
pH (potential of hydrogen): the symbol for hydrogen ion concentration, a scale of numbers which expresses exactly how acid or alkaline something is.
pheomelanin: the natural hair pigment responsible for the yellow and red tones in hair.
pincurl: a strand of hairs organised into a flat ribbon form, and wound into a series of continuous untwisted circles within circles.
pityriasis: the correct name for dandruff, the overproduction of epidermal scales.
plait: intertwining of hair strands to form a braid.
plastic cap: a cap used to cover the hair to help retain moisture and body heat, and so speed up processing.
porosity: the ability of the hair to absorb liquids.
porosity test: test to check the porosity of the hair, check the condition of the cuticle.

porous: full of pores, able to absorb liquids.
processing time: the period of time required for a chemical action upon the hair to achieve the desired result.
psoriasis: a non-infectious skin condition that is sometimes seen on the scalp, characterised by thick silvery scales.

quaternary ammonium compounds: group of chemicals with germicidal properties which can be used as detergents and conditioners. They have a positive charge; cetrimide is a good example.

reverse pincurling: the placing of open pincurls in alternate rows, in clockwise and anticlockwise directions.

sebaceous glands: the oil glands attached to the hair follicle. They secrete sebum directly into the hair follicle.
sebum: the oily secretion of the sebaceous gland; helps lubricate and waterproof the skin.
sectioning: dividing the hair into separate parts, or panels.
sectioning clip: a clip used to secure sections of the hair.
sensitivity: being easily affected by chemicals, resulting in a skin reaction.
shampoo: to wash the hair with detergent and water or the name given to a soapless detergent used to clean the hair.
shingling: using the scissor over comb technique to cut hair short in the neck region.
soapless shampoo: a shampoo that contains a synthetic detergent rather than a soap. Almost every shampoo used today is soapless.
sodium hydroxide: a caustic chemical, commonly called lye, used in a number of hair relaxers. It can also be used to dissolve hair in blocked basins and drains.
spiral winding: winding the hair from roots to points.
split ends: damage to the ends of the hair which results in splitting along the length of the hair; the correct term is *fragilitis crinium*.
spongy: porous.
stand-up curl: an open pincurl which stands up from its base producing volume at the roots.
static electricity: the term used to describe the build up of a charge on the hair, caused by friction when brushing or combing hair, especially when newly dried.
steamer: a machine used to produce moist, moving heat.
stem direction: the part of the pincurl that determines its direction.
symmetrical: evenly balanced.

tail comb: a comb, half of which is shaped into a slender, tail-like end.
tapering: removing length and bulk from the hair using either scissors or a razor on wet hair.
terminal hair: the coarse hair found on the scalp and other areas of the body after puberty (beard, underarms and pubic region).

ultra-violet: the invisible rays present in sunlight that promote tanning of the skin.
under-directed: the placing of a roller on a base which is equivalent to twice the diameter of the roller and the same length as the roller so that it sits on the lower part of the base. This produces minimum volume.

vellus hair: the soft downy hair found on the body.
vertex: the top, or crown, of the head.
vibro: an electrical machine used to give mechanical massage.
virgin hair: this usually refers to hair which has not been previously chemically processed, but in the case of black hair it refers to hair which has not been previously relaxed or straightened.

Index

Afros, 118–21
alpha-keratin, 135–6

backbrushing, 153–4
backcombing, 152–3
basins, 39–42
beta-keratin, 135–6
brushes, 62–6

chignons, 192–9
children, 130–32
client
   communication, 24–38
clippers, 74
club cutting, 107–8
combs, 66–8
conditioners, 175–81
cutting, 105–33

design analysis, 84–92

effleurage, 184
electrical appliances, 43–57
extensions, 206–9

face shapes, 85–7
finger waving, 137–42
first aid, 19–22

French pleat, 200–2
friction, 185

gels, 169–70

hair, 1–5
hair chemistry, 5–7
hair clips, 57–9
hair shapers, 75–6
hairlines, 120–22
hairsprays, 166–8
high frequency, 187–90
hygiene, 9–12

Mad Mats, 62
massage, 182–6
Molton Browners, 61, 156–8
mousses, 168–9

oil treatments, 181–2

partings, 102–3
petrissage, 184
pH, 7–8
pincurls, 142–5
plaiting, 202–6
pli, 136–7
preparation, 93–103

razors, 75–80
reception, 25–30
retailing, 35–6
Rik-Raks, 61
rollers, 59–60, 145–51

salon layout, 16–19
salon organisation, 211–28
salon safety, 12–16
setting, 134–58
setting lotions, 164–6
scissors, 68–74
shampooing, 95–102
shampoos, 98–100
shingling, 116–17
spiral curlers, 60
split ends, 117–18

tapering, 108–9
tapotement, 185
telephone technique, 27–8
texturising hair, 113–15
thinning hair, 111–13
treatments, 173–91

water sprays, 62
wrap round, 155–6

vibro, 186